Ethics Primer

of the

American Psychiatric Association

This book was supported by a grant from the American Psychiatric Foundation.

Ethics Primer

of the

American Psychiatric Association

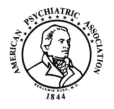

Published by the
American Psychiatric Association
Washington, D.C.

Note: The findings, opinions, and conclusions of this report do not necessarily represent the views of the officers, trustees, or all members of the American Psychiatric Association. Each report, however, does represent the thoughtful judgment and findings of the committee of experts who composed it. These reports are considered a substantive contribution to the ongoing analysis and evaluation of problems, programs, issues, and practices in a given area of concern.

Manufactured in the United States of America on acid-free paper
04 03 02 01   4 3 2 1
First Edition

American Psychiatric Association
1400 K Street, N.W.
Washington, DC 20005
www.psych.org

Library of Congress Cataloging-in-Publication Data
American Psychiatric Association.
    Ethics primer of the American Psychiatric Association.
        p. ; cm.
    Prepared by members of the Ethics Committee of the American Psychiatric Association.
    Includes bibliographical references and index.
    ISBN 0-89042-317-2 (alk. paper)
    1. Psychiatric ethics—United States. I. American Psychiatric Association. Ethics Committee. II. Title.
    [DNLM: 1. Ethics, Medical—United States. 2. Psychiatry—standards—United States. WM 62 A512e2001]
    RC455.2.E8 A47 2001
    174'.2—dc21

                                                                00-058662

British Library Cataloguing in Publication Data
A CIP record is available from the British Library.

Contents

Contributors. vii

Introduction: Role of the APA in Developing and
Enforcing Psychiatric Ethics ix
   David S. Wahl, M.D.

Introduction for Psychiatric Residents xiii
   Daniel S. Polster, M.D.

1

Boundary Violations. 1
   Peter B. Gruenberg, M.D.

2

Children, Adolescents, and Families. 11
   William Arroyo, M.D.

3

Geriatric Populations 23
   Lesley Blake, M.D.

4

Involuntary Hospitalization 27
   Richard D. Milone, M.D.

5

Managed Care 33
   Donald G. Langsley, M.D.

6

Confidentiality 39
Lawrence Hartmann, M.D.

7

Gifts 45
Daniel S. Polster, M.D.

8

Duty to Report Colleagues Who
Engage in Fraud or Deception 51
Mary Marshall Overstreet, M.D., J.D.

9

Ethics of Emergency Care 57
Beverly J. Fauman, M.D.

10

Ethics and Forensic Psychiatry .65
Robert M. Wettstein, M.D.

11

Consultations and Second Opinions 75
Gary S. Weinstein, M.D.

APPENDIX

The Principles of Medical Ethics With Annotations
Especially Applicable to Psychiatry, 2001 Edition 79

Index 93

Contributors

American Psychiatric Association
Ethics Committee

Except where otherwise indicated, all contributors are associated with the American Psychiatric Association Ethics Committee.

William Arroyo, M.D.
Sherman Oaks, California

Lesley Blake, M.D.
Chair, Illinois Psychiatric Society Ethics Committee,
Glenview, Illinois

Carol Davis
Director, APA Office of Ethics and Professional Responsibility,
Washington, D.C.

Beverly J. Fauman, M.D.
Ann Arbor, Michigan

Peter B. Gruenberg, M.D.
Beverly Hills, California

Lawrence Hartmann, M.D.
Cambridge, Massachusetts

Donald G. Langsley, M.D.
Evanston, Illinois

JoAnn E. Macbeth, J.D.
Legal Counsel, Crowell & Moring LLP,
Washington, D.C.

Richard D. Milone, M.D.
Harrison, New York

Wade C. Myers, M.D.
Gainesville, Florida

Mary Marshall Overstreet, M.D., J.D.
Dexter, Maine

Daniel S. Polster, M.D.
APA Committee of Residents and Fellows Representative,
University Heights, Ohio

David S. Wahl, M.D.
Lakewood, Colorado

Gary S. Weinstein, M.D.
Assembly Liaison,
Louisville, Kentucky

Robert M. Wettstein, M.D.
Pittsburgh, Pennsylvania

Introduction

Role of the APA in Developing and Enforcing Psychiatric Ethics

David S. Wahl, M.D.

"Should I accept a patient's invitation to a party?" "Can I release sensitive information about my patient without the patient's consent?" "Can I treat a close friend of a patient?" "Is it OK to tell a patient that I, too, have had a depression?" "Is it OK to co-treat a patient with someone I know to be less than competent?" "A local newspaper asked for my opinion about a politician's well-known habitual drinking. Can I give it?" "Was it unethical to get angry with my patient?" "Can I give a psychiatric opinion about someone I've never examined?"

None of these questions calls to mind a clear "yes" or "no" answer. These questions all require careful balance among the clinical circumstances of the patient, the community and culture in which treatment is provided, the training and values of the psychiatrist, and the ethical code of our profession. With each dilemma, there are ethical principles that help the ethical physician fashion the best response. Oftentimes the principles conflict with one another, and the psychiatrist must make a judgment based on his or her weighing of the competing principles. The essence of an ethical resolution to an ethical dilemma is the process by which the principles are weighed. This process of self-inquiry and debate is the tradition upon which today's ethical principles are built—and continue to evolve.

"Can I solicit money from my patients to help with my new on-line Web page?" "I want to create a commercial videotape of depression using my patients but not tell them of my plans for distribution...is that OK?" "Is it possible to ethically arrange a sexual relationship with my patient?" "Can I release records about deceased patients without their permission?"

Here, the ethical questions lend themselves more clearly to definitive answers, based on ethical principles. Indeed, each represents more of a moral principle of behavior than an ethical conflict. And again, you find clear guidance in seeking those moral imperatives by referring to the age-old traditions of the ethical principles of the medical profession.

From Hippocrates, through the many turns and interpretations over the centuries, to current renditions of medical ethics, we have inherited a rich legacy of principles, guidelines, and even rules to help us. Each generation of physicians has yielded new insights into those principles, and, thus, we live with an evolving set of guidelines and of conduct.

The most recent iteration of that tradition is *The Principles of Medical Ethics With Annotations Especially Applicable to Psychiatry* (American Psychiatric Association [APA] 2001). This manual, first published by the APA in 1973 and updated regularly, is based on *The Principles of Medical Ethics by the* American Medical Association (AMA). All editions of the *Principles* for psychiatry begin with the following preamble (with a shorter statement for pre-1980 editions):

> The medical profession has long subscribed to a body of ethical statements developed primarily for the benefit of the patient. As a member of this profession, a physician must recognize responsibility not only to patients but also to society, to other health professionals, and to self. The following Principles, adopted by the American Medical Association, are not laws but standards of conduct, which define the essentials of honorable behavior for the physician. (APA 2001)

Simply put, *The Principles of Medical Ethics* for psychiatry is a listing of guidelines and standards to guide us (see Appendix of this book). The reader who journeys through this primer will gather a richer appreciation for the wisdom and subtleties of those guidelines and principles.

Nevertheless, we are faced with the ever present realities of members of our profession who violate these principles. Section 2 states, "A physician shall deal honestly with patients and colleagues, and strive to expose those physicians deficient in character or competence, or who engage in fraud or deception" (APA 2001), calling on us as a profession to identify and, when necessary, discipline members who behave unethically. Although licensing boards, hospital review committees, and medical societies oftentimes tackle these issues, as psychiatrists, we have chosen to establish a system through the APA and its district branches to respond to complaints of potentially unethical conduct.

On the basis of fundamental principles of fairness and comprehensiveness, the APA, through the voluntary commitment of local ethics committees in each district branch, seeks to fully and confidentially investigate all applicable ethical complaints, conduct full and fair hearings, and decide appropriate sanctions when a finding of ethical misconduct is determined. Sanctions range from reprimand to suspension, or even expulsion from the APA and the district branch, with an overriding interest in rehabilitation and education. Throughout the process, complainants and accused members are treated with dignity and respect as the peer review process unfolds. To learn about the details of that process, interested physicians can inquire through their local district branches or the APA Office of Ethics and Professional Responsibility. (*The Principles of Medical Ethics With Annotations Especially Applicable to Psychiatry* includes a section that describes the APA's procedures for handling complaints of members' unethical conduct.)

The trends of reviewed conduct within and outside of ethical principles assist the profession in illuminating the evolving nature of these ethical principles. From case material from each disciplinary proceeding, we learn about how changing practice, societal values, and individual choices affect the application of ethical principles. The fluid interplay of these factors reemphasizes the ever changing nature of ethical principles. Many vignettes in the chapters of this primer have emerged through the formal proceedings of the APA Ethics Committee, although they are disguised to preserve confidentiality.

Another important process that helps psychiatrists develop ethical standards involves less formal endeavors, such as clinical consultations. By way of letters of inquiry, phone calls, or curbside consultations, psychiatrists are ever searching for input from one another about ethical dilemmas. All the contributors to this primer are recognized as community and national leaders in the field of psychiatric ethics and hence are exposed to a wealth of clinical dilemmas through the informality or formality of consultation. This is perhaps the richest source of information for the material presented here.

This primer helps the psychiatrist, whether in training or in established clinical practice, to develop a structure for addressing the myriad ethical and moral choices that present themselves to our field. Each chapter specifically addresses concrete ethical dilemmas in contemporary psychiatric practice with clinical vignettes and ethical principles to help guide the ethical physician in seeking ethical solutions to those dilemmas that are commonplace in our work. From boundaries to work within managed care settings, from confidentiality to unique circumstances around treatment of special populations, the reader should find this book helpful in delineating an ethical approach to the patient.

Most important among the goals of the editor and contributors to this volume is to encourage the reader to begin discussions with colleagues and friends about the questions raised in these pages. If the vignettes and chapters serve only to answer questions with a "yes" or "no," then the richest of our ethical traditions will themselves be violated. In the final analysis, our code of ethics is an organic, dynamic, and ever evolving set of standards, and this primer will successfully serve that process by stirring you, the reader, to carry on in that tradition of inquiry, debate, and examination.

Reference

American Psychiatric Association: The Principles of Medical Ethics With Annotations Especially Applicable to Psychiatry. Washington, DC, American Psychiatric Association, 2001

Introduction for Psychiatric Residents

Daniel S. Polster, M.D.

It has truly been a pleasure to spend the last two years collaborating with the American Psychiatric Association Ethics Committee on the development of ethics education materials for psychiatric residents. This primer represents one aspect of that project, one that we hope will take its place as essential reading for every psychiatric resident for years to come.

Many of us feel that too little time is devoted to teaching physicians in all medical specialties about ethics pertinent to that discipline. Indeed, beginning in medical school, finding room to teach an ethics course is challenging alongside the constantly expanding knowledge base. In some instances an ethics course might be sacrificed to make room for the more concrete science of medicine. When ethics courses are designed, they rarely focus on issues specific to any one field but, rather, on those pertinent to all medical students: end-of-life issues, confidentiality, and many others.

Yet psychiatry—without sounding too self-absorbed—is special. The practice of psychiatry is different from other fields of medicine. The general ethics issues taught in medical school continue to apply, but the doctor–patient relationship in psychiatry is much more complex than in other disciplines. As such, multiple ethical issues arise that other physicians may not routinely face. Boundary violations? Duty to warn? Involuntary hospitalization? These issues may not arise to the same degree outside of psychiatry and are sometimes ignored by the rest of the medical world.

So when is a psychiatrist to learn these principles? Residency is the time when these lessons should be taught and enforced so that any psychiatrist is well versed in them by the time he or she goes into practice. The reality, however, is that residency—like medical school—often devotes too little time to teaching about psychiatric ethics. Our constantly evolving psychopharmacological armamentarium keeps residents constantly busy learning the latest in medications, whereas financial pressures and service obligations limit the amount of time that faculties have to teach courses on ethics. Once again, the ethical issues pertinent to psychiatry may be sacrificed in young residents. And once those residents have completed their education and are in practice, it may be too late. The rest of the profession and society expect them to know the principles and to behave in an ethical manner.

The foregone conclusion, then, is that ethics education in psychiatry must take place during the residency. Or no ethics education may take place at all. We have developed this primer to help guide residents through many of the complex ethical issues that psychiatrists may face every day. Although this primer may not guide you through every ethical challenge that you may face in your career, these chapters are a starting point. We want you to be aware of standard ethical principles, but also to begin to think in a way that will help you solve future ethical dilemmas. In addition, we hope that this primer will be a springboard for further discussions among your residency programs and an educational tool that you can use to complement any existing ethics training you may have.

Last, we hope this primer is fun and interesting to read, with some clinical vignettes and examples to bring the principles themselves into a real-life clinical context. This primer should not be limited to residents only, but may be helpful to medical students and early career psychiatrists alike. In fact, we hope you find it helpful throughout your careers and wish you all the best of luck in them.

1

Boundary Violations

Peter B. Gruenberg, M.D.

The Frame and Its Boundaries

The relationship between the psychiatrist and the patient is special. This unique relationship has been evolving over the past 150 years. It started in the nineteenth century when our forebears, the Alienists, cared for patients in the large public and private asylums, hospitals, retreats, sanatoriums, and prisons. With the insights of Freud and others, more psychiatrists began to see patients privately, and the principles derived from dynamic psychotherapy and psychoanalysis greatly influenced the relationship that psychiatrists had with their patients. This distinct relationship was not only unique as between people in general, it was also unique even among other physicians. Even so, the guiding ideals can be traced to the early behavioral and ethical codes of the ancient physicians. The Hippocratic oath lays the groundwork for the overarching principle of altruism. It suggests that the physician practice in a manner that benefits the patient and not gossip about and not exploit the patient.

In attempting to consolidate the ancient ideas of altruism and the modern ideas of unconscious memories, affects, and motivations, Langs (1977) proposed the concepts of the therapeutic frame and Gabbard and Lester (1995) have illuminated the concepts of therapeutic boundaries.

Langs advised us that psychotherapy occurs within a frame that sets the boundaries of the therapeutic relationship. One part of the frame is composed of the mutually agreed upon constants of the relationship. These constants include the absence of physical contact, confidentiality, constant place of the meeting (e.g., the doctor's office),

1

payment of a constant fee, and length and frequency of the sessions. The other part of the frame is composed of the human elements of the therapeutic situation and include nonjudgmental acceptance by the therapist, an effort to understand the meaning of communications and behaviors, relative anonymity of the therapist, the agreement by the patient to say whatever comes to mind, abstinence from inappropriate gratifications, offering appropriate gratifications, offering concern and efforts to understand, interpretations of unconscious conflicts as they become apparent, and a particular focus on understanding the interaction between psychiatrist and patient (Gabbard and Lester 1995).

Psychoanalytic thinking has given us abundant boundaries to consider. For example, there are boundaries between the conscious and the unconscious; the psychic and the somatic; the ego, the id, and the superego; the patient and the doctor; the patient's unconscious and the doctor's unconscious; the me and the not-me; sleep and wakefulness; the self and the object; and the internal object and the external object. In ethical terms, there are (or should be) boundaries between, for example, the professional relationship and a social relationship, the professional relationship and a sexual or romantic relationship, the professional relationship and a business relationship, and the professional relationship and a caretaking relationship by the patient. Any passage over the boundary between the professional relationship and any of the other classes of relationships can be called a *boundary crossing*. A serious boundary crossing may be termed a *boundary violation*. This chapter draws attention to the presence of boundaries and the possibilities of boundary crossings and violations and, by doing so, tries to minimize them.

⌒〜

Boundary Crossings

The psychiatrist's office is on the twentieth floor of an office building. The mail slot has been jammed for several days. The doctor asks a patient to mail a letter for him on the way out, saving him a long round-trip on the elevator. *That is certainly a boundary crossing between the professional relationship and caretaking relationship. Is it also a boundary violation? That all depends. Is the envelope a payment to the telephone company or a statement to another patient? The issue of confidentiality comes up. Is it a communication to a brokerage house? What fantasies are stimulated by such an envelope?*

A patient asks for an aspirin for a headache. The doctor happens to have a bottle for her own use. *Does giving the aspirin cross a boundary? Does it violate a boundary?*

A patient mentions that a company he knows of is going to be taken over by a larger company, and its stock will surely go through the roof. *May the doctor inquire as to the name of the company? May he quietly buy some of the stock? What are the boundary issues here?*

Sexual Boundary Violations

The oldest specific admonition for physicians involves abstaining from sexual involvement with patients. Hippocrates, in the fifth century B.C.E., wrote:

> Into whatever houses I enter, I will go into them for the benefit of the sick, and will abstain from every voluntary act of mischief and corruption; and, further from the seduction of females or males, of freemen and slaves.

Whether Hippocrates was aware of transference or countertransference is unknown. He was, however, keenly aware that a sexual relationship was incompatible with the trust that was necessary for a physician to inspire. Various other portions of the Hippocratic oath have been discarded (e.g., cutting for the stone), but this particular item has remained and is the one admonition that all physicians and almost all laypersons recognize.

Thus, for the past 2,500 years, sexual activity with a patient has been forbidden by our own oath. It was not until 1973 that the American Psychiatric Association first published *The Principles of Medical Ethics With Annotations Especially Applicable to Psychiatry*, which included the phrase: "Sex with a current patient is unethical. Sex with a former patient is almost always unethical" (American Psychiatric Association 1973, p. 4).

In 1993 the American Psychiatric Association Board of Trustees approved a revision of that annotation. In all iterations of the *Principles* published since then, the statement is now absolutely unequivocal and reads, "Sexual activity with a current or former patient is unethical" (American Psychiatric Association 2001, Section 2, Annotation 1).

But it is more complicated than that. Sexual activity with the mother (or father) of a child patient is similarly unethical. This would apply to close relatives and caregivers of patients as well.

The overarching principle is that we must have only one kind of relationship with a patient—that is, a doctor–patient relationship. Dual relationships are fraught with danger for patients and for ourselves. Further, we understand that it would be impossible for a patient to give informed consent to such a relationship because of unconscious transferences that are bound to occur. Sexual involvement, then, is an exploitation of a patient's primitive feelings, and thus an exploitation of the patient.

The Slippery Slope

In a large majority of cases involving sexual contact with patients and that are brought to ethics committees, a familiar pattern emerges. The sexual activity does not occur in a vacuum. Sex does not happen in an unguarded moment of mutual passion. There are hints and precursors. Often, we hear of seemingly innocuous boundary crossings. A cup of coffee together. A ride home. A hug. A squeeze of the hand. A longer hug. A kiss on the cheek. A kiss elsewhere. A shared scheme involving the psychiatrist. Any one of these boundary crossings could be, in and of itself, innocent enough. But when they become part of a pattern, one must become alarmed. As some of these behaviors occur, there is a shift away from the exclusive professional relationship toward a dual relationship that might include the professional relationship as well as a social or romantic relationship.

Nonsexual Boundary Crossings and Violations

Sexual boundary violations are relatively easy to describe and to exhort against. Nonsexual boundary violations (e.g., crossing the boundary between the professional relationship and the social, business, personal, caregiving, or pseudoparental relationship) are more difficult to describe—and giving strict rules is more difficult.

Self-Disclosure

In the past decade or two there has been a move away from the absolute prohibition of any type of self-disclosure. That absolute prohibition was derived from classical psychoanalytic technique in which the anonymity of the analyst provided a blank screen upon which the analysand could project elements from his or her own unconscious. Even psychiatrists not practicing analysis recognized that telling patients about themselves sometimes had the effect of burdening the patient with the doctor's own problems. This tended to add a separate component to the professional relationship, an additional element of the patient becoming a caregiver. Further, some disclosures may be heard by the patient in ways that are unintended by the psychiatrist. For example, a psychiatrist who, with the intent of strengthening rapport with a patient, says "Yes, I can understand how you feel. I never got along with my father either." The patient may hear this in a way that suggests that the doctor is even more flawed than the patient feels himself to be, thus decreasing the rapport.

Yet, there is increasing discussion in analytic as well as in nonanalytic circles about how much and what kind of self-disclosure is appropriate and under what circumstances. The decisions are complex and involve a thorough knowledge of the psychodynamics of the patient and the conscious and unconscious meanings of such disclosure. So, although the frame is changing and the use of self-disclosure is increasing, this situation is fraught with potential problems. The best advice continues to be: *When in doubt, don't.*

Certain types of self-disclosure are certainly inappropriate under any circumstances. These include disclosing the psychiatrist's fantasies concerning the patient, especially those of a sexual nature. Therapists' dreams in general should not be discussed, especially if they have a sexual content and most especially if they involve the patient.

On the other hand, some types of self-disclosure are now felt to be essential. If the doctor has become ill and there is the likelihood that he or she may become disabled or incapacitated, the patient should be told, so that the patient can be helped to decide if continuing with that doctor is in the patient's best interests. This speaks to the issue of patient autonomy and informed consent, both laudable ethical principles. Further, if the psychiatrist has an obvious injury or illness, it is probably better to inform the patient of the nature of the injury rather than allow the patient's fantasy to run away. However, under certain analytic circumstances, self-disclosure of this sort may be contraindicated.

Gifts

The subject of gifts has attracted a considerable amount of attention and is the subject of Chapter 7 of this primer. Other medical specialists are often given gifts, and no particular harm seems to result. But psychiatrists are committed to understand all communications, both verbal and nonverbal. The giving and receiving of gifts is certainly the type of communication that deserves our attention. Does the patient feel that a gift must be given? How does the patient get such an idea? Is the psychiatrist's office filled with wrapped presents during the holidays? If so, what does that tell the next patient who comes through the door? Many psychiatrists feel it is appropriate to accept small gifts at the holiday season with little or no interpretation. Expensive or suggestive gifts should be declined with whatever explanation or interpretation is appropriate.

Physical Contact

In the not too distant past, psychiatric residents were prohibited from touching their patients in any way. If some contact became necessary, for example, taking the pulse or blood pressure, another resident was asked to do it. Such prohibitions are quite rare now, but thoughtful precautions should be taken before touching a patient. One of the most common problems is that the patient might experience the touch in a way that is quite different from the way the doctor offered it. An avuncular hug from a kindly senior psychiatrist may be experienced as the prelude to a sexual or romantic shift. Certain patients are more inclined to such misinterpretations than are others. Everything considered, it is best to avoid physical contact. Yet problems can occur when touching is avoided.

> A male patient was in analysis with a male analyst. When the psychiatrist opened the waiting room door to bring the patient into the consulting room, the patient would extend his hand to shake the psychiatrist's hand. This practice had gone on for many months. One day the psychiatrist opened the waiting room door and saw the patient, who had a bad cold, wiping his nose with his hand. As the patient extended his hand, the doctor pulled back his own hand. The patient perceived this as a severe rejection of himself (as opposed to the germs), and the doctor suffered through many hours of diatribe and vituperation. *In retrospect, perhaps the daily handshake should have been examined earlier for its meaning of acceptance by the doctor for the patient.*

> A male psychiatrist treated a female patient for several years in weekly psychotherapy. Numerous seriously traumatic events befell the patient during that time, and the psychiatrist was supportive. They had gone through a lot together. It came time to terminate the treatment, and the termination was worked through. At the last session, both got

up, and the doctor opened the door for the patient. As the patient went by the doctor, she stopped and gave him a spontaneous hug. The doctor froze and did not reciprocate. The patient instantly recognized the doctor's predicament and laughed as she pointed out that she certainly felt freer than he did. He felt bad that, indeed, he did not feel free to give an appropriate human response.

Confidentiality

Confidentiality, a major issue in the containment of boundaries, is discussed in Chapter 6 of this primer.

Financial Relationships

Financial relationships with patients clearly form a separate and distinct class of relationship and, with the exception of the circumstances surrounding the agreed-upon fee, are to be avoided. One should not hire one's patients or their relatives to do work, even if the work to be performed benefits both the doctor and the patient.

> A psychiatrist hires a patient to do some electrical work on his house. *Should the fee be based on the hourly rate of the psychiatrist or of the electrician? If the rates are different, one or the other may be resentful. If there is a problem with the work, should the doctor bring it up with the patient during the session or call him in the evening? If a dispute occurs, how can it be resolved without interfering with the treatment?*

> A patient invites her psychiatrist to become a partner in a business venture. The doctor is flattered and accepts. The doctor takes on more and more responsibility and buys more and more stock until she controls the board and the company. The patient feels preempted by the psychiatrist and brings a lawsuit. *This can have serious consequences for the treatment!*

A barter arrangement is tempting to consider for the patient who cannot afford the psychiatrist's regular fee. However, there are a number of problems here. First, unless both parties to the barter arrangement report the value of the services received as income, the barter is illegal. In addition, numerous problems may occur, as with the financial relationship cited earlier. How will the barter be constructed? One hour of therapy for one hour of baby-sitting? One hour of therapy for 20 hours of baby-sitting? What happens if the work is not acceptable? Is this grist for the mill, or should it be settled in a different way? Who has the power? Who needs to please whom and why? It is certainly a lot cleaner for the patient to do his or her work and pay the doctor for the doctor's work.

Information

As noted earlier, using information such as data on a financial deal crosses the boundary between professional relationships and business relationships and should be avoided. Other sorts of information that may become available in a treatment situation should similarly not be taken out of the office or used in any way. This would include, in addition to stock tips, information about the patient's financial status; information about the financial or other aspects of the patient's family, friends, and associates; and political information. These boundaries merge with the area of confidentiality, which proposes that whatever information is brought forward in the office stays in the office. As Hippocrates advised:

> Whatever, in connection with my professional practice or not in connection with it, I see or hear, in the life of men, which ought not to be spoken of abroad, I will not divulge, as reckoning that all such should be kept secret.

Autonomy

In the past few decades, there has been a shift in medical ethics away from paternalism and toward autonomy. The doctor does not always know best, and further, an informed and competent patient ought to be able to make his or her own decisions. Good clinical practice alone would dictate that fostering adult behavior in adults is better than infantilizing them. It is not uncommon for psychiatrists to be quite directive with some patients. One must be certain that this directiveness is in the best interests of the patient and does not fulfill some need of the psychiatrist. As an example, suggesting that a patient go into the field of medicine may be in the interests of the patient, but it also may derive from the doctor's wish to control or to have a disciple. It may be a displacement from the doctor's wish that his or her own child go into medicine.

Influences

Similarly, the psychiatrist should avoid influencing the patient in any way not directly relevant to treatment goals. This would obviously include attempts to persuade the patient in religious matters, in matters concerning sexual orientation, and in political circumstances. From time to time, psychiatrists feel a moral duty to address these concerns with their patients. If one cannot resist such temptations, supervision should be sought or the patient transferred to another psychiatrist.

Recently there has been a temptation to engage patients in social and political matters that might aid patients generally. Extreme care must be taken to ensure that it is not the doctor's own interests that are at work.

Our nonpsychiatric medical colleagues are occasionally involved in fund-raising activities on behalf of their hospital, medical school, or charity. It is not uncommon for them to solicit contributions from their grateful patients. Psychiatrists should avoid participating in such activities, because doing so often relies on unresolved transference feelings and thus exploits the patient. If a former patient wishes to show his or her gratitude by making an unsolicited gift to an organization, such a patient should be directed to the development specialist at the organization or to an otherwise uninvolved colleague who will assist with the donation.

References

American Psychiatric Association: The Principles of Medical Ethics With Annotations Especially Applicable to Psychiatry. Washington, DC, American Psychiatric Association, 1973

American Psychiatric Association: The Principles of Medical Ethics With Annotations Especially Applicable to Psychiatry, 2001 Edition. Washington, DC, American Psychiatric Association, 2001

Gabbard G, Lester E: Boundaries and Boundary Violations in Psychoanalysis. New York, Basic Books, 1995

Langs R: The Therapeutic Interaction: A Synthesis. New York, Jason Aronson, 1977

2

Children, Adolescents, and Families

William Arroyo, M.D.

 Salient issues that have greater relevance in the psychiatric care of children as opposed to that of adults include contexts of development, family, and treatment coercion. (The word "children" will be used throughout this chapter to refer to both children and adolescents, unless otherwise specified.) The ongoing developmental changes in the biological, psychological, and social domains have broad implications for both treatment of the patient and conduct of the psychiatrist. The ethical approach to evaluating and treating children is virtually always in the context of the family, the primary unit of the child's environment. At times another key participant such as a teacher may be instrumental in providing the child treatment. In one of the remaining frontiers of psychiatry, infant psychiatry, there are virtually always at least two people, i.e., mother and infant, in treatment.

Developmental issues will dictate other aspects of the care provided. A young child, for example, will not generally understand abstract concepts that may be discussed with parents because of the child's level of cognitive development.

Children are generally reluctant or involuntary participants in the treatment process. The parent desires some change in the child's behavior or thoughts and hopes that the psychiatrist can accomplish this goal. Children are generally much less informed about psychiatric care than their parents are and oftentimes do not appreciate their parents'

The author deeply appreciates the assistance provided by Diane Schetky, M.D., in preparation of this chapter.

desire to have them change. Thus, engagement of the child in the early phase of psychiatric treatment often requires different strategies from those that would ordinarily be used with adults. These strategies may vary depending on developmental factors. Some adolescents, for example, may be defiant and provocative participants early in the process, whereas a 5-year-old girl may immediately play with the available toys in the office.

This chapter will highlight those issues that residents and other psychiatrists encounter in the early part of their careers in working with children. These include informed consent, psychopharmacology, confidentiality, psychotherapy, boundary issues, and hospitalization. Confidentiality and boundary issues are also discussed in Chapters 6 and 1, respectively.

⌒

Informed Consent

Informed consent by the patient is both an ethical and a legal necessity of providing psychiatric care. *Consent* refers to the legal authority to give permission. *Assent* refers to the child's affirmative agreement to participate in the treatment. Obtaining assent from a child becomes more important with increasing age of the child.

An important part of the strategy to engage a child and a family is to explain what activities constitute psychiatric care. The information provided to a parent must, of course, be modified for a child depending on the child's age. However, the same information may be given to a parent as to an older teenager with adult cognitive abilities. Most adults will easily understand the goals of talk therapies but may need more detailed explanations, for example, about the use of play in the treatment of younger children.

Parents hold the right to give informed consent for the provision of psychiatric care to their children under the age of 18, with some exceptions, of which some are noted below. It is generally assumed that when a parent brings in a child for a psychiatric evaluation or treatment, consent is implied. Although this may, in fact, be true, informed consent provided by a patient has evolved into a formal process. Specially designed forms completed by patients (or their parent if the patient is under 18) signify their possession of the necessary information about the proposed care, alternative treatments, and risks versus benefits. Completion of such forms indicates their voluntary acceptance of such care and their competence (or intellectual capacity) to make binding decisions about their lives.

While parents have the legal authority to give informed consent for medical care to their children under the age of 18, in special circumstances, state statutes may designate legal authority for giving consent to others (Behnke et al. 1998). Such exceptions include situations involving emergencies, emancipated minors, and adults who have had their parental rights legally curtailed or modified, among others. In addition, state laws vary in certain instances, e.g., abortion, transplants, and psychopharmacology. However, statutes relevant to informed consent do not preclude obtaining assent from a child about the care to be provided.

Children of Divorced Birth Parents

An increasingly common challenge for psychiatrists who treat children of divorced birth parents is the issue of legal custody. A parent with legal custody has the legal authority to give informed consent relating to psychotherapy and the administration of psychotropic medications. Both parents of a child may each have legal custody in most states. It behooves every psychiatrist who treats children of divorced parents to identify the parent with legal custody. The involvement of both birth parents (and sometimes both stepparents) in the treatment of a child may be clinically and ethically indicated. It is unethical to submit to family court a professional opinion on the parenting capability of each of the divorced birth parents without interviewing each of them. A psychiatrist must insist on interviewing each of the parents before agreeing to provide an opinion.

Children in Foster Care

Children in foster care are another special group for whom identification of legal authority can be challenging. This authority varies widely from state to state. For example, in some states the dependency court judge has the legal authority, and the assigned caseworker may be able to exercise the consent. In California the legal authority rests with dependency court for psychotherapy—but for psychotropic medication, the authority rested with the birth parent until very recently, when a law was passed that removed such legal authority from birth parents.

The legal authority for psychotropic medication is now under the purview of the dependency court judge. In addition, special procedures and policies have been developed to process requests for the use of psychotropic medications with foster care children in California. Most states do not require similar special requests by physicians for treatment of foster care children with psychotropic drugs.

Emancipated Minors

Emancipated minors generally have the same legal authority to give informed consent that adults have. The determination of "emancipation" is not always easy. Emancipated minors are children of minority age, usually at least age 14 and under age 18, who willingly live apart from parents or guardians with their consent or acquiescence (not necessarily written). These minors can provide their own informed consent for treatment purposes. In addition, emancipated minors manage their own financial affairs and do not derive their primary income from criminal activity. Minors are also emancipated if married or on active duty in the armed forces. Under other special circumstances, some states grant emancipated minors legal authority to give informed consent for mental health services (however, not necessarily for psychotropic medication) at the age of 12.

Psychopharmacology

The increasingly broad range of psychotropic drugs that are routinely used with adults are being used to treat children. However, the relative lack of a substantial database related to indications, benefits, and risks of the use of psychopharmacological agents with children (as opposed to adults) should compel psychiatrists to use a judicious approach to prescribing psychotropic agents to children; such an approach may include more frequent medication follow-ups. Parents often raise questions regarding the Food and Drug Administration's approved uses of psychotropic medication versus unlabeled uses; this topic may be integrated into the informed consent discussion with patients and their families.

An important developmental issue relevant to this area is metabolic rates. Younger children (prepubertal) often metabolize and excrete drugs faster than do adolescents and adults; children therefore may require higher doses per body weight than the other age groups. However, developmental vulnerability to toxicity is evident in the use of certain medications, including tetracycline, known to induce tooth discoloration; aspirin, which may cause Reye's syndrome; valproic acid, which may precipitate hepatic failure or increase the risk of developing polycystic ovary disease; and hexachlorophene, which can have an adverse effect on myelin.

The potential developmental risks of long-term effects of a particular mental disorder versus the risks of long-term use of psychotropics must be considered by parents, the treating psychiatrist, and, often, the child.

A frequent clinical challenge is reconciling the desire of the parent to administer medication to effect changes in behavior versus the child's unwillingness to take the prescribed medication. Some psychotic adolescents, for example, will refuse to take antipsychotic medication on a routine basis despite their parents' great desire for them to do so. Some parents have become so insistent that their child take the medication that they devise secret strategies to make their child comply. One such parent of a 17-year-old patient with schizophrenia would place medication in milk or juice at mealtime without the teenager's knowledge to ensure administration of medication; the patient's psychotic thinking went into remission. This strategy backfired when the patient refused any medication, using as a basis for the decision the recent absence of psychotic thinking and anger at the parents triggered by the disclosure of the secret administration. I had previously engaged the parents in lengthy discussions about the risks related to this method of medication administration. Psychiatrists at times may need to guard against participation in similar circumstances that are ethically and clinically problematic.

Nonpharmacological interventions should be given initial consideration for virtually all preschool children. Some, however, may briefly require a psychotropic medication. School-age children may be at less risk for problems due to psychotropic agents than are preschool children and generally will assume more responsibility for the administration of their medication. Although many children at ages 10–12 years are able to engage in abstract thinking according to Piaget's cognitive developmental theory, many have the capacity to express an opinion about their care by about age 7. Therefore, it would be prudent for a psychiatrist to attempt to obtain assent from children as young as age 7 for whom psychotropic medication is prescribed.

Adolescents will often be the final decision maker as they assume increasing autonomy regarding the self-administration of psychotropic medication. Therefore, psychiatrists must educate such teenagers about the benefits and risks of medication. Psychiatrists should closely monitor this group for side effects relating to weight gain and sexual function, which are often normal developmental concerns even without psychotropic medication. Self-image may be another normal concern of a young adolescent. Peer pressure and the stigma of being "a mental" will also challenge any good psychiatrist.

Confidentiality

Confidentiality is an ethical cornerstone of psychiatry. The tenet of confidentiality breeds the patient's trust of the psychiatrist, trust that is essential to the psychiatrist's work. The slightest of breaches may undermine the care of a patient. This issue becomes a bit more complex when working with children than in the treatment of adults (Morrissey et al. 1986; Schetky 1995; U.S. Department of Health and Human Services 1999).

Adolescents, for example, will rarely share their sexual history, substance abuse history, and even their multitude of depressive symptoms with their parents but will do so with a trustworthy psychiatrist, who is perceived as providing a safe environment to discuss these personal issues. Parents who complain that their teenager will not discuss anything with them are hopeful that this type of rapport will develop. Many parents are also eager to have the psychiatrist disclose these details. The dilemma psychiatrists encounter relates to the importance of honoring confidentiality with the patient, who is virtually always identified as the child.

Therefore, it is imperative to discuss confidentiality in a clear fashion with the child and family at the outset of treatment. I generally initiate this discussion by asking if the family members in attendance are familiar with this topic, how it might apply to their specific case, and the legal exceptions (discussed further in this section). I have found in general that 1) a parent agrees not to insist that the psychiatrist give specific details of sessions with, for example, the adolescent; 2) a parent agrees not to review (or obtain a copy of) the medical record for this purpose; and 3) a parent sometimes agrees not to "harass" the adolescent about these details.

These guidelines are rarely contested by the child and family, in large part because the guidelines do not preclude the child from sharing the details of the sessions with parents. These guidelines also do not preclude the psychiatrist from urging the child to share certain information with the parents or from obtaining the child's assent to have the psychiatrist share certain information with the parents. I may negotiate with the child and family at the outset to periodically give the parents a general update of the child's progress, as frequently as after each session; this update should be provided with the child present.

For children below the age of 7 or 8, maintaining confidentiality is important, but it tends to have a different clinical significance than it has with older children and adolescents. Young children are less apt to insist that information not be disclosed to, for example, parents; these children will generally disclose unlimited details of their sessions to their parents. Nonetheless, it is prudent to discuss with young children what the treating psychiatrist hopes to share with the parents before doing so, especially if the psychiatrist has assured the young child about "absolute" confidentiality. In a different circumstance, the treatment of infants dictates that maintaining confidentiality pertains to the mother—or caretaker—and infant dyad. The ethics principle of confidentiality generally applies to the actions and information shared during the course of providing care to a patient, whether care is in the context of a family session or an individual one.

Exceptions to Protecting Patient Confidentiality

There are several exceptions in many states to a psychiatrist's protection of patient confidentiality. These include the threat of a patient's harm to self, the threat of a patient's harm to others, and a suspicion that a patient has been a victim of child abuse. The patient's intent to harm him- or herself is generally the least difficult for psychiatrists to report to parents or authorities. Conversely, a young resident or psychiatrist may be riddled with anxiety and ambivalence the first few times of reporting a patient's intent to harm others or a suspicion of child abuse. Regarding a patient's intent to harm others, notifying a potential victim of possible harm by one's patient is a challenge for most practitioners; sometimes the local authorities will help facilitate this task. In wrestling with the obligation to report a suspicion of child abuse, a common misconception among young (or veteran) psychiatrists is their perception that the act was not truly child abuse. Our ethical and legal obligation, however, is not to determine whether or not abuse actually occurred but to report a suspicion of abuse; the actual determination is made in the judicial system. In reporting a suspicion of child abuse, another common fear is that the patient and family will drop out of treatment; this result is common, and equally common is that the family resumes psychiatric care elsewhere, albeit under court direction.

Nonclinical Factors Affecting Confidentiality

The thoughts and feelings that a patient shares in confidence with the psychiatrist are often entered into a medical record. However, access to these records is not determined solely by the patient or the treating psychiatrist.

Thus, the following may often conflict with the principle of confidentiality: state statutes, state regulations, policies of third-party payers related to disclosure of patient information, and the pervasion of information technology. Most states give legal authority to parents to either review or obtain a copy of the medical record; children generally do not have the legal right to do so. (However, some states make exceptions to accessing medical records. In California, the exceptions in which a child has a right to obtain a copy of his or her medical records occur when the child has the legal authority to give consent for care, such as in the case of an emancipated minor. In addition, a parent or an emancipated minor in California can obtain a copy of a record when a potential detriment to the patient–doctor relationship and potential physical or emotional harm to the child patient exist.) Third-party payers such as managed care plans almost always require varying levels of disclosure of medical records, ostensibly for billing and other administrative purposes. In addition, the influx of information technology, including electronic medical records, has triggered a new series of debates regarding confidentiality and privacy of medical records. In Congress and in state legislatures, maintaining privacy of medical records is a hotly contested issue.

⌒

Psychotherapy With Children and Families

The initial experience of treating children and their families often varies widely among psychiatrists in training. Child and adolescent psychiatric rotations often begin during the second or third year of general psychiatric training. A certain level of comfort and self-confidence has been achieved by the time a resident begins to see children. Residents who have their own children or who have rotated through pediatrics are initially generally more comfortable communicating with children than those who have not. Many residents enjoy the interactions and rotation, whereas others clearly acknowledge their ambivalence and lack of self-confidence in working with children and families. Communicating with young children or adolescents can be very challenging, yet very rewarding.

Setting the goals of psychotherapy with children varies from the standard used with adult patients. Since the child rarely seeks psychotherapy on his or her own, this exercise must generally be conducted in conjunction with the child and parents.

The treatment of a child may present unique ethical challenges. For example, young children who are hospitalized and therefore separated from their families frequently evoke strong feelings of protection and caretaking in newly trained psychiatrists. Similarly, adolescents who have antagonistic relationships with their parents may share a list of conflicts that are historically identical to those a young psychiatrist recently had with his or her own parents. In some instances, these conflicts are ongoing, and the patient's parents may be erroneously blamed by the psychiatrist as he or she identifies with the patient. This countertransference may potentially undermine the delivery of competent intervention. The novice psychiatrist must be able to distinguish between his or her own needs and those of the patient. If this is too difficult, the ethical decision would be to consult with one's clinical supervisor, and subsequent transfer of care may be optimal.

The family as the "patient" may present other ethical challenges. Many parents believe that a child's behavior is under the sole control of the child who fails to appreciate the "ideal" modeling provided by the parents and perhaps other family members. However, there may be instances when the psychiatrist's opinion, based on a thorough evaluation, parallels that of the adolescent, for example, when the adolescent claims the parents are the ones who need to change. It is then the psychiatrist's ethical responsibility to convey this to the parents in a manner that invites them to adopt a new perspective conducive to effective intervention. Then parents may acknowledge, for example, that their constant shouting and arguing trigger similar behavior among their children—the idea originally presented by the adolescent identified by the parents as having "the problem." Subsequently, the psychiatrist might focus on teaching family members nonaggressive strategies to resolve their differences.

⌒

Boundary Issues

Boundary violations with children are varyingly contratherapeutic and, in certain circumstances, illegal. It is atypical for a psychiatrist to provide psychotherapy to a child who does not evoke a broad range of thoughts and emotions either initially or later during the course of psychotherapy. Some may include anger, joy, a tugging at the psychiatrist's parental instincts, and even sexual arousal. These feelings and thoughts are almost always normal responses. The challenge for the psychiatrist is to acknowledge them, to refrain from acting on these urges, and to assess them in the context of the child, family, and optimal clinical care.

One of the more egregious boundary violations is having a sexual encounter with a child patient. Virtually all acts of sex by a psychiatrist with a patient are an attempt by the psychiatrist to meet the psychiatrist's needs or desires. Such exploitation can take the shape of many forms; skin-to-skin contact is not a prerequisite for such exploitation. For example, a rapidly maturing, pubertal 11-year-old girl who is infantilized for a long duration by her parents and has a history of sexual abuse by a male may repeatedly seek close physical proximity to the male psychiatrist. The psychiatrist will need to clearly structure the young adolescent, acknowledge any sexual arousal on his part, and proceed with psychiatric care in an ethical fashion.

Very young children tend to be more impulsive and may naturally seek physical comfort from a caring and attentive adult. Setting structure primarily for clinical reasons should be considered.

Boundary violations must also be considered with respect to the child's family members. Socializing or becoming intimate with a family member may seriously jeopardize the psychiatric care provided to a child and therefore is unethical.

Spending some time with one's patient outside the traditional settings of hospitals and outpatient facilities is encouraged in virtually all training programs, either during the child and adolescent rotation of a general psychiatric training program or during the more intensive child and adolescent residency. This may take the form of conducting individual psychotherapy during a walk in a park or to the local fast-food restaurant in an urban area. Away from the typical clinical setting, psychiatrists should develop an awareness of the boundary issues in these circumstances. First, confidentiality cannot be ensured if the possibility exists of running into, for example, a classmate of the patient. Someone may eavesdrop on the conversation while strolling in the public venue. Second, the selection of the patient with whom to conduct such treatment is also important. For example, selecting a patient from an inpatient service on which the child is a risk for elopement could have dire consequences (including medicolegal ones), as well as ethical implications of competence. Third and last, one must guard against socializing during such activity because socializing with a patient undermines effective treatment. Examples of potential boundary violations are rarely discussed with trainees. Such potential violations should, however, be considered in deciding whether or not a psychiatric trainee or psychiatrist should conduct psychotherapy outside traditional settings. Residency directors should be encouraged to teach about potential boundary violations.

Hospitalization of Children

The frequency and duration of hospitalizing children have dramatically decreased during the past decade, in large part because of the penetration of managed care throughout the health care industry. In addition, medical necessity criteria, which are virtually always based on adult populations, have limited applicability for some children who require hospitalization. Medical necessity criteria rarely incorporate acknowledgment of differences between adults and children. This recent pendulum swing to rare and short hospital stays has threatened the financial viability of teaching hospitals and the integrity of psychiatric training programs across the nation; significant downsizing and actual closures of teaching hospitals have not been uncommon in the recent past. For-profit and not-for-profit teaching hospitals have been compelled to develop other strategies to stay financially afloat.

Residents in teaching facilities have not been exempt from these pressures. A decision to hospitalize a child at a facility with low occupancy rates and serious financial problems, primarily or in part to "save" the teaching facility, may be unethical for various reasons, including a conflict of interest for the psychiatric trainee who decides that his or her need to maintain the training program outweighs the clinical indication for a less restrictive level of care. Similarly, the relative lack of beds in some states may compel a physician to deny hospitalization despite the clinical indication to the contrary. A novice resident or young psychiatrist should consult with a supervisor (or colleague) not only in regard to a decision to hospitalize but also in regard to the relevant ethical considerations.

Conclusions

Ethical standards of conduct relevant to the psychiatric treatment of children are determined primarily by developmental and family factors. Many standards, such as confidentiality and structuring boundaries, are time-honored principles of medical ethics that predate modern psychiatry. Statutes and case law, which frequently change, also strongly influence the psychiatric care of children. Periodic review and updates of all of these factors are imperative to the provision of good care.

References

American Academy of Child and Adolescent Psychiatry: Code of Ethics. Washington, DC, AACAP, 1982

Behnke SH, Preis JJ, Bates RT (eds): The Essentials of California Mental Health Law. New York, WW Norton, 1998

Morrissey JM, Hofmann AD, Thrope JC (eds): Consent and Confidentiality in the Health Care of Children and Adolescents—A Legal Guide. New York, Free Press, 1986

Schetky DH (ed): Ethics. Child Adolesc Psychiatr Clin N Am 4(4), 1995

U.S. Department of Health and Human Services: Confidentiality of mental health information: ethical, legal, and policy issues, in Mental Health: A Report of the Surgeon General. Rockville, MD, U.S. Public Health Service, 1999

3

Geriatric Populations

Lesley Blake, M.D.

Aging is not a disease; it does not necessarily imply physical and intellectual deterioration. Simply being older in no way implies that a new, or looser, code of ethics is applicable. The principles of medical ethics that apply to younger patients also apply to those patients in older age groups. However, many medical problems—dementing illnesses in particular—are much more common with advancing age, and that, together with an often associated decline in social and economic conditions, may lead to an increase in ethical issues for the psychiatrist who treats older patients.

While some ethical and value issues are unique to the psychiatric care of the elderly, many are shared with other age groups in psychiatric practice. For example, efforts at cost containment and the rationing of medical services are impinging deeply on psychiatric patients, many of them elderly. Psychiatric consultants at nursing homes are more frequently asked by nursing staff to evaluate patients, only to find that the patients' insurance will not cover psychiatric care. At this stage, psychiatrists are left with the ethical dilemma of either providing care for which they will not be reimbursed but for which they are liable, or letting the patient's psychiatric problem go untreated. If this happened with just a few patients, it would not cause much difficulty; but when such patients begin to constitute a significant number of consultation referrals, it becomes more of a problem. Working with older patients, we are faced with ethical quandaries on a daily basis. Some are more straightforward than others; some seem insurmountable—but with a clear understanding that we must do the best for our patients, be thoughtful of ethical issues at all times, and try to do the right thing, most issues can be resolved to a comfortable extent.

Confidentiality

Confidentiality is a cornerstone of psychiatric practice. With older psychiatric patients, there is often the ethical dilemma of the need to share important medical and psychiatric information with third parties (other physicians, family members, caregivers, and insurance companies). A conflict may arise between preserving the patient's autonomy and avoiding potential harm to the patient or society. Although one's primary duty to the patient may be to preserve confidentiality, in the interest of patient or societal safety, sometimes the best course of action involves divulging information. This should always be done on a case-by-case basis, with confidential consultation with an ethics expert if necessary. Because a patient is elderly does not imply that the usual need for confidentiality no longer exists.

Competence and Consent

Psychiatrists are often asked to make judgments about a cognitively impaired patient's capacity to make decisions about his or her medical care. Again, a dilemma arises from preserving the patient's autonomy and avoiding harm. Discussions about the patient's decision-making capacity need to focus on the medical issues at hand and not on the patient's global abilities. This often needs to be carefully explained to the patient's family and other treating physicians, since the patient may be capable of making decisions about medical care but not about financial dealings. The psychiatrist also should try to identify and decrease factors that may diminish the patient's decision-making capacity. These could include factors such as depression, sleep deprivation, metabolic imbalance, and medication side effects. The ethical issue in determining competence involves obtaining all information available and using that information to determine the balance between exercising paternalism and encouraging autonomy—and between coercion (forcing patients into treatment or financial decisions against their will) and neglect (allowing patients to refuse treatment or financial help despite a great known risk attached to this).

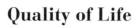

Quality of Life

Often with the combination of advanced age, medical illnesses, and cognitive impairment, the patient's family and physicians may see little quality in the patient's life, and therefore little value in continuing it. The patient may also voice wishes to end his or her life. The ethical difficulty that the psychiatrist faces in this situation is the need to look at the situation from the patient's perspective, rather than from the desires of the psychiatrist, the family, and other physicians. The psychiatrist should also look at ways of maximizing the patient's quality of life given the medical, economic, and time constraints. Often, small changes in the patient's environment, treatment regimen, or caregiver can improve the patient's quality of life. When the psychiatrist helps to identify these factors, alterations can frequently be made; these can significantly improve the patient's outlook.

Abuse and Neglect

Physicians have the ethical and legal obligation to ascertain and report cases of elder abuse and neglect. In many cases, this clearly benefits the patient, but often reporting abuse and neglect is a difficult issue. Patients often depend on the abusers for support and may prefer to risk further abuse, rather than be forced to move from their home of many years into a nursing home. Together with the psychiatrist's legal obligation in these matters comes the ethical obligation to determine whether the patient's own desires can be met by working with the family, legal system, social service agencies, and other involved health care professionals. The risks, benefits, and alternatives to institutionalization and legal action against caregivers need to be carefully examined in light of the patient's expressed wishes and needs.

Use of Restraints

The greatest predictor of the use of restraints in acute and long-term care facilities is cognitive impairment. Ethical dilemmas can develop from decisions that limit patients' freedom of movement against their wishes or in situations where patients cannot make their wishes known. Federal guidelines prohibit the use of restraints for staff convenience, but they are still widely used for the protection of the patient or those around the patient. The decision to use restraints over the patient's objections always requires careful consideration of the risks and benefits and should never be an automatic decision, since it always decreases the patient's autonomy. Whenever possible, ethically working toward environmental and behavioral interventions should always be considered before ordering restraints. Creating a safe environment for patients has been shown to significantly decrease the prevalence of injuries, when compared with an environment where restraint is used regularly.

Research

While there has been a definite need to test the safety and effectiveness of psychiatric treatments in the elderly, the ethics of research on this population continues to need monitoring. Issues related to informed consent in cognitively impaired patients, the use of double-blind studies when approved treatment alternatives are available, the risk of coercion, and the involvement of nursing home populations all present ethical dilemmas. Working closely with patients' families and nursing home staff—and with primary care physicians, institutional review boards, and ethics committees, if available—helps to clarify these issues. However, the final ethical responsibility still lies with the psychiatric researcher, who must ensure that the benefits always outweigh the risks.

Conclusions

Despite the myriad ethical dilemmas encountered on an almost daily basis, working with older patients is very rewarding. Seldom are the issues straightforward or clear-cut, and many will involve consultation with family members, other treating physicians, social service agencies, and the legal system. However, as psychiatrists, we are uniquely qualified to be true patient advocates, trying to maximize our patients' autonomy while protecting them from harm, intent on doing the right thing at all times.

4

Involuntary Hospitalization

Richard D. Milone, M.D.

Few issues in the field of mental health evoke more controversy than involuntary commitment and treatment. Involuntary hospitalization becomes a meeting place for several ethical principles, including some that conflict with one another. These include utilitarianism, beneficence, autonomy, and informed consent, to name a few. This chapter presents these ethical principles as equal bases on which to choose or not choose involuntary treatment for a patient. Below, the principles observed in supporting and opposing involuntary treatment are introduced, followed by a discussion of coercion and recent legal developments that provide context for this issue.

Ethics Principles for Involuntary Treatment

The paragraphs below present opposing ethical viewpoints on involuntary treatment. While the statutes for involuntary hospitalization vary from state to state, it is generally acknowledged that this treatment decision requires two elements: (1) the presence of a severe mental disorder that deprives the individual of the capacity to make treatment decisions; and (2) the likelihood of harm to self or to others. Choosing involuntary hospitalization for a patient who does not meet both of these criteria would be unethical, and often, illegal.

In Favor of Involuntary Treatment

Those who support involuntary treatment for the mentally ill likely uphold the utilitarian principle—that is, through treatment, lessening or completely removing the barrier that mental illness forces onto an individual will eventually give that individual a better life. This view holds that the temporary deprivation of physical liberty is justified by the eventual good of returned health.

Similarly, the principle of beneficence directs physicians and others to care for individuals incapable of caring for themselves. Supporters of beneficence believe that involuntary hospitalization restores autonomy to the mentally ill through treatment. Further, the argument is made that society has the right to limit an individual's freedom when necessary to protect others from serious harm.

Opposed to Involuntary Treatment

Those opposed to involuntary treatment support the principles of autonomy and libertarianism. Proponents of these principles attest that an individual has a right to exist independently without control by others. In this view, forcing someone into hospitalization is an act of paternalism—that is, "Father [or the authority figure] knows best, and you should do whatever he tells you to do." Further, from these perspectives, liberty is such an important value to society that it transcends all other values—and involuntary hospitalization is a clear infringement of a person's liberty. One passage frequently cited by libertarians to support their position is John Stuart Mill's treatise *On Liberty*:

> [The] only purpose for which power can be rightfully exercised over any member of a civilized community, against his will, is to prevent harm to others. His own good, either physical or moral, is not a sufficient warrant. He cannot rightfully be compelled to do or forbear because it will be better for him to do so, because it will make him happier, because, in the opinions of others, to do so would be wise, or even right. (Mill 1912, p. 15)

⌒⌐

Involuntary Treatment and the Issue of Coercion

Can treatment that is coerced be effective and does coercion have any place in medicine, either psychiatry or general medicine? In its publication *Forced Into Treatment: The Role of Coercion in Clinical Practice*, the Group for the Advancement of Psychiatry stated: "Coercion, persuasion, suggestion and direction are legitimate dimensions of both parenting and treatment, but they require careful scrutiny, and their use demands that the clinician be scrupulously reflective" (Group for the Advancement of Psychiatry 1994, p. 2).

Bloch, Chodoff, and Green quoted the same document by the Group for the Advancement of Psychiatry in their comprehensive text *Psychiatric Ethics* (Bloch et al. 1999). Regarding the place of coercion in the treatment of the mentally ill, Bloch et al. quoted the Group for the Advancement of Psychiatry as follows:

> As we examine these forced-treatment solutions, we found repeatedly that initial coercion can lead to greater freedom....as we researched and studied the exceptions to the original premise that coercion is antithetical to treatment, we began to view coercion not in terms of presence or absence, but in terms of degree and source....Voluntary and forced treatments lie on a continuum with different elements working to strengthen motivation. We believe that optimism in these forced-treatment situations can be justified. We encourage psychiatrists to provide such treatment when appropriate to help the patient progress from a posture of defiance, to compliance, to alliance. (Bloch et al. 1999, p. 431)

In recent years, the argument by Thomas Szasz and others that mental illness is a myth (Szasz 1961) has, for the most part, subsided. New and effective treatments, particularly the advent of safe and effective antidepressant and antipsychotic medications, have improved the lot of the patient and shortened hospitalization. The report in December 1999 from the Surgeon General of the United States (U.S. Department of Health and Human Services 1999) points especially to the efficacy of psychiatric treatment. The Surgeon General's report defines mental disorders as legitimate illnesses that respond to specific treatments, just as other health conditions respond to medical intervention. The question in recent times is less one of whether involuntary hospitalization should take place, but, more, under what circumstances should involuntary hospitalization occur.

Involuntary Hospitalization and the Law

A psychiatrist's decision to use involuntary treatment is made within the parameters of current state law on the issue. Therefore, it is important to remain informed about one's state laws on this topic and any changes that may occur. State legislatures appear to be moving toward a middle ground that meets the treatment needs of the severely mentally ill, while at the same time preserving their legal rights. Below, a discussion on the government powers that these laws reflect.

The law under which involuntary hospitalization may take place is perhaps best expressed in the preamble to the Constitution of the United States. Two powers are identified: the police power and the *parens patriae* power. First, for the benefit of society, governments are responsible for protecting each citizen from other persons' injurious actions. This is called the police power, and the issue here is dangerousness of the individual and protection of citizens from the individual in question. Second, governments have the power and the duty to protect individuals who cannot do so themselves. This is the principle of *parens patriae*, when governments are the parent of last resort for each citizen. Here, the needs of the individual are of concern, and the issue is a need for treatment. It is important to remember that the *parens patriae* power is a benevolent one regarding the patient, the individual who cannot protect herself; that is, government is responsible for the care of a disabled citizen as loyally as a parent would care for a child.

Shift Toward Dangerousness Standard

The current trend in civil commitment moves away from the *parens patriae* standard toward criteria that make dangerousness to self or to others the principal determinant of eligibility for involuntary hospitalization. Coincidental with this shift has been a marked limitation of the psychiatrist's power to commit an individual to involuntary hospitalization without court approval, and patients have been granted procedural protection similar to that granted to criminal defendants.

Stavis, writing for the Treatment Advocacy Center, reported a celebrated case that demonstrates the shift away from *parens patriae* and toward the dangerousness standard (Stavis 1989). The case, which occurred in New York in 1987, involved Ms. Billie Boggs (a pseudonym for her real name).

> Ms. Boggs was a 44-year-old woman who lived on the public sidewalk of an affluent New York City neighborhood. She was frequently seen by personnel from emergency psychiatric services and was described by them as dirty and disheveled, speaking in sexually oriented rhyme, exposing herself, and smelling of excrement. She also exhibited other erratic behavior such as tearing up money and urinating on it.

New York City Health and Hospitals Corporation sought to have Ms. Boggs involuntarily committed for care and treatment because such treatment was essential for her welfare. This effort by New York City Health and Hospitals Corporation was vigorously opposed on behalf of Ms. Boggs by the New York Civil Liberties Union, which contended that her main problem was homelessness. Both parties agreed that commitment of Ms. Boggs must meet standards showing that the alleged mental illness is potentially dangerous or likely to result in harm to the individual or others. New York City Health and Hospitals Corporation successfully proved that Ms. Boggs was more than merely dysfunctional and proved that her judgment was impaired due to her mental illness. But, at least initially, it was not able to establish her dangerousness, and so she returned to the streets essentially untreated.

Stavis further explained:

[The] Boggs case illustrates that patients who could truly benefit from mental health treatment will be more unlikely to obtain help because the illness also causes a denial or an unawareness of its own existence. This is unfortunately not consistent with the parens patriae power under which the government is supposed to behave as a parent in helping those who do not have competent decision making ability and who cannot cope with a major aspect or function of life even if there isn't a true imminent danger. It was very arguable whether Ms. Boggs was a danger to herself or others. After all, she existed for more than a year and a half on the streets of Manhattan without sustaining any significant injury or causing any direct harm to anyone. She sustained a pattern in her life including obtaining food, having a primitive sanitary system and having clothing. (Stavis 1989, p. 3)

The effect of this trend away from the *parens patriae* power of government toward the "dangerousness" or police power is to relegate government's benevolent intervention only to those instances in which harm can be foreseen. In a climate in which "dangerousness" prevails as the determinant for involuntary hospitalization, the benefit of merely restoring an individual's mental health, or returning to an individual the ability to care for himself or herself, becomes insufficient reason for the government to invoke its serious power of civil commitment.

Outpatient Involuntary Treatment

In late 1999, New York State enacted legislation that provides for assisted outpatient treatment and certain mentally ill individuals who, in view of their psychiatric history and current circumstances, are unlikely to survive safely in the community without supervision. The new law, commonly referred to as "Kendra's law," was named after a young woman who died after being pushed in front of a New York City subway train by a mentally ill person who had failed to take the antipsychotic medication prescribed for his illness. The law establishes a procedure by which a court can order outpatient treatment as described in a written treatment plan previously approved by the court (New York Mental Health Hygiene Law, Section 9.60).

References

Bloch S, Chodoff P, Green S (eds): Psychiatric Ethics, 3rd Edition. New York, Oxford University Press, 1999

Group for the Advancement of Psychiatry: Forced Into Treatment: The Role of Coercion in Clinical Practice. Washington, DC, American Psychiatric Press, 1994

Mill JS: On liberty, in The World's Classics, Introductory. London, Oxford University Press, 1912

New York Mental Health Hygiene Law, Section 9.60 (Kendra's Law, Assisted Outpatient Treatment "AOT")

Stavis PF: Involuntary Hospitalization in the Modern Era: Is "Dangerousness" Ambiguous or Obsolete? Treatment Advocacy Center, 2300 N Fairfax Drive, Suite 220, Arlington, VA 22201, 1989

Szasz TS: The Myth of Mental Illness. New York, Dell, 1961

U.S. Department of Health and Human Services: Mental Health: A Report of the Surgeon General. Rockville, MD: U.S. Department of Health and Human Services, Substance Abuse and Mental Health Services Administration, Center for Mental Health Services, National Institutes of Health, National Institute of Mental Health, 1999. S/N 017-024-01653-5.

5

Managed Care

Donald G. Langsley, M.D.

What Is Managed Care?

Under managed care, budgets rather than professional guidelines set
the standards for medical practice, while managed care organizations
(MCOs) make large profits and pay huge salaries to their executives.
Since the world moved into third-party payment, treatment decisions
are made by those who pay the bills. *The doctor examines the patient
and establishes a treatment plan*, but some other person who has never
seen that patient—another physician, a nurse, social worker, psychologist, or even a clerk with no medical training—decides whether the patient receives the recommended treatment. Furthermore, although
these decisions are sometimes based on guidelines known to the physician treating the patient, more often they are not. Although doctors
would like to use guidelines supported by scientific medicine, often
they do not know who developed the guidelines for approving treatment decisions and have no input into guideline revisions. In some circumstances, physicians have an obligation to initiate appeals on behalf
of their patients if they consider the MCO decision to be contrary to the
patient's best interests. Yet if an attending physician disagrees with the
MCO decision and appeals, the original MCO decision stands. Even
when MCO actions harm patients, doctors cannot sue the MCO because it is protected by a federal law called the Employee Retirement
Income Security Act of 1974 (ERISA).

Patients trust that their doctors will come to their aid—this trust
is the very basis of the doctor–patient relationship. As part of the process of giving informed consent, physicians should disclose all treatment alternatives, regardless of cost and regardless of whether the

MCO pays for that particular treatment. However, when physicians want to explain to the patient what alternative treatments are scientifically appropriate, many MCOs "gag" the doctor from discussing alternatives not approved by the MCO. In addition, patients in acute distress who would like to go to a nearby hospital emergency room for immediate attention cannot do so because most MCOs require advance approval to obtain emergency services. The tradition of a patient choosing his or her doctor applies only when the desired doctor is a member of the MCO panel; if the doctor is dropped from the panel, the patient must find a new doctor from the approved list. In most cases, the right to see a specialist applies only when the patient is first seen by a primary care physician in the MCO.

Physicians must place the patient's interests ahead of their own, including financial remuneration. However, MCOs often compensate physicians with capitation fees that give doctors a financial advantage to withhold treatment. Instead, financial incentives should be based on demonstrated quality of care rather than on the quantity of services.

⌒

Effects of Managed Care on Medical Practice

All of the criticisms above have been leveled at the managed care industry, although not all apply to every managed care plan. Because decisions are made outside of the doctor–patient relationship and are based on cost to the plan, vigorous and even violent complaints have been made about the managed care industry. Some of those complaints have been heard by government, courts, legislators, or by the MCOs themselves; and some of those practices (e.g., the requirement to see a primary care physician for referral to a specialist) have been modified over the past year or two. However, there continues to be widespread dissatisfaction with the managed care system, and physicians have asked themselves whether they can ethically practice medicine under such a system.

The criticisms apply to general health plans operated by MCOs, but many of these MCOs have turned over the responsibility for mental health treatments to a system of "carve outs" for mental illness and behavioral health. The rationale has been that specialized systems are needed for mental health services. Psychiatrists usually deal with the specialized behavioral health MCOs, and criticisms of these organizations have been similar to those of the general managed care system.

Psychiatrists who deal with managed care organizations should use guidelines that will permit them to be comfortable with the ethical standards they follow in these transactions. Such guidelines have been developed by the American Medical Association, the American Psychiatric Association, and experts on ethics in managed care, such as Sabin. These particular guidelines are delineated below for reference.

Guidelines Developed by the American Medical Association[1]

1. The duty of patient advocacy is a fundamental element of the physician–patient relationship. Physicians must place the interests of their patients first.
2. When managed care plans place restrictions on care, the following principles should be followed:
   a. Allocation guidelines that restrict care and choices (beyond the cost–benefit judgments made by physicians) should be established at a policymaking level, not on an ad hoc basis by individual reviewers.
   b. Physicians must advocate for any care they believe will materially benefit their patients.
   c. Physicians should be given an active role in contributing their expertise to any allocation process. Guidelines should be reviewed regularly and updated.
   d. Adequate appellate mechanisms for both patients and physicians should be in place.
   e. Managed care plans must adhere to the requirement of informed consent that patients be given full disclosure of material information.
   f. The physician's obligation to disclose treatment alternatives is not altered by any limitation in the coverage provided by managed care.

---

[1]Council on Ethical and Judicial Affairs, American Medical Association 1995, pp. 330–335

g. Physicians should not participate in any plan that encourages or requires care at below minimum professional standards.

3. Financial incentives are permissible only if they promote the cost-effective delivery of health care and not the withholding of medically necessary care. Health plans and other groups should develop financial incentives based on quality of care.

⌒

Guidelines of Practice for Managed Care Reviewers

These guidelines were approved by the American Psychiatric Association Board of Trustees, October 18, 1999.

The American Psychiatric Association defines these guidelines of practice as applicable to psychiatrists functioning as medical directors and medical reviewers working for MCOs. Psychiatric reviewers working in medical review, precertification, retrospective review, and necessity of ancillary service utilization and diagnostic test utilization are bound by sound clinical principles and judgment. Psychiatrists who render judgments that deny a patient the care recommended by their treating psychiatrist or other mental health clinicians should do so only after obtaining a full and complete medical understanding of the facts and the situation of the patient by reviewing appropriate records, tests, and procedures and consulting with the patient's treating physician.

Reviewers should not selectively entertain data to support their decisions while eliminating contradictory data from discussions and consideration. Their decision should be based on sound medical principles embraced by the medical community and should not be arbitrary or capricious. If patients are seriously ill and there is a dispute concerning judgment that relates to the patient's immediate safety and security, the attending physician's judgment should prevail. The managed care medical directors or reviewing physicians should understand that some courts have ruled that some reviewers are making medical decisions related to patient care when they override the judgment of the treating physician or disallow recommended care.

Psychiatric reviewers should only practice in systems that have a prompt and competent system of decision appeal. In reviewing medical necessity for treatment and precertification, reviewers must

(1) use standards appropriate to the community where the patient resides when determining the medical needs of the patient; and (2) make determinations based upon "reasonable" need and the likelihood that the patient will benefit from appropriate treatment.

The reviewer's job is to ascertain the appropriateness and necessity of recommended medical treatment, not simply to curtail costs. The reviewer should never refuse or reduce needed treatment. The American Psychiatric Association affirms the position of the American Medical Association that no managed care director or reviewer should receive compensation based on bonuses obtained by the reduction or elimination of care, nor should they receive compensation from hold-backs based on performance of disallowal of care. Managed care reviewers should treat both patients and their colleagues with dignity and respect. They should provide specific written reasons for the disallowal of requested treatments and procedures and include information about the appeals process. Reviewers, like treating physicians, are subject to legal and ethical sanctions for misconduct.

In summary, medical directors and managed care reviewers should consider themselves physicians first, dedicated to the constructive use of resources in an attempt to provide assistance to patients rather than deny care. They should work with treating physicians as colleagues and neither override nor disallow decisions without a sound medical basis that is then communicated in writing.

Sabin's Credo for Ethical Managed Care in Mental Health Practice[2]

1. As a clinician, I am dedicated to caring for my patients in a relationship of fidelity and at the same time, to acting as a steward of society's resources.
2. As a clinician, I believe it is ethically mandatory to recommend the least costly treatment unless I have substantial evidence that a more costly intervention is likely to yield a superior outcome.

---

[2]Sabin 1994, pp. 859–860

3. In my stewardship role, I need to advocate for justice in the health care system, just as in my clinical role, I need to advocate for the welfare of my patient.
4. If a potentially beneficial intervention does not meet the explicit public standards for third-party coverage in a just system, as a clinician I believe the ethical course is to withhold the intervention and to discuss the situation openly with my patient.

Conclusion

Managed care has afforded major ethical challenges to the psychiatrist. The comments and cited ethical standards in this chapter may offer some guidelines to the practitioner.

References

Council on Ethical and Judicial Affairs, American Medical Association: Ethical issues in managed care. JAMA 273:330–335, 1995

Sabin JE: A credo for ethical managed care in mental health practice. Hosp Community Psychiatry 45:859–860, 1994

6

Confidentiality

Lawrence Hartmann, M.D.

T he basic rule to follow about patient confidentiality is that psychiatrists should keep all patient material confidential at all times. This powerful and fundamental ethics principle sometimes clashes with other ethics standards. However, a psychiatrist should follow this rule unless there is a very strong ethical reason not to do so. Even if you think there is a reason to diverge from this rule, be careful and thoughtful about any exceptions you make to confidentiality, and from time to time, read about specific relevant areas of ethics or get consultation on the subject—or both.

Good medical care requires a high level of confidentiality. Respect for confidentiality is supported by long tradition, the Hippocratic oath, and *The Principles of Medical Ethics With Annotations Especially Applicable to Psychiatry* (American Psychiatric Association 2001; see Appendix of this primer). For psychiatric patients, because of the widespread stigma and many cultural contexts of mental versus physical illness, confidentiality is even more important than in most areas of medicine (American Psychiatric Association Committee on Confidentiality 1987).

Section 4, Annotation 1 of the *Principles of Medical Ethics With Annotations Especially Applicable to Psychiatry* (hereinafter *Principles*) defines psychiatric medical records and comments on the necessity for confidentiality: "Psychiatric records, including even the identification of a person as a patient, must be protected with extreme care. Confidentiality is essential to psychiatric treatment. This is based in part on the special nature of psychiatric therapy." The *Principles* go on to note that this is an era of growing concern about "the civil rights of patients and the possible adverse effects of computerization, duplication equipment, and data banks" (Section 4, Annotation 1). These advances in technology may provide relatively easy access to data, but "because of the sensitive and private nature of the information with which the psychiatrist deals, he/she must be circumspect in the information that he/she chooses to disclose to others about a patient. The welfare of the patient must be a continuing [dominant] consideration" (*Principles*, Section 4, Annotation 1).

Section 4, Annotation 2 of the *Principles* deals with how and when confidential information may be released: "A psychiatrist may release confidential information only with the authorization of the patient or under proper legal compulsion. The continuing duty of the psychiatrist to protect the patient includes fully apprising him/her of the connotations of waiving the privilege of privacy. This may become an issue when the patient is being investigated by a government agency, is applying for a position, or is involved in legal action. The same principles apply to the release of information [about a patient] to medical departments of government agencies, business organizations, labor unions, and insurance companies. [For example,] information gained in confidence about patients seen in [college] student health services should not be released without the students' explicit permission." A parent or legal guardian should give authorization in the case of a young child or unemancipated minor. Informed consent and competence to give consent must both be present and the authorization to give information should usually be framed narrowly and in time-limited ways.

Clinical information is often used in teaching or in publishing articles in professional journals. Section 4, Annotation 3 of the *Principles* states that "clinical and other materials used in teaching and writing must be adequately disguised in order to preserve the anonymity of the individuals involved." Section 4, Annotation 10 of the *Principles* also deals with this issue, stating that "with regard for the person's dignity and privacy and with truly informed consent, it is ethical to present a patient to a scientific gathering, if the confidentiality of the presentation is understood and accepted by the audience." Section 4, Annotation 11 of the *Principles* also touches on this issue, stating that "it is ethical to present a patient or former patient to a public gathering or to the news media only if the patient is fully informed of enduring loss of confidentiality, is competent, and consents in writing without coercion."

There is a similar ethical responsibility regarding information derived from a consultation. Section 4, Annotation 4 of the *Principles* states that "the ethical responsibility of maintaining confidentiality holds equally for the consultations in which the patient may not have been present and in which the consultee [was or] was not a physician. In such instances, the physician consultant should alert the consultee to [the consultee's] duty of confidentiality."

Because of the type of fantasies or historical information which may be revealed, the psychiatrist must be cautious about what to disclose, even when permission is granted. Section 4, Annotation 5 of the *Principles* states that "ethically, the psychiatrist may disclose only that information which is relevant to a given situation. He/she should avoid offering speculations as fact. Sensitive information such as an individual's sexual orientation or fantasy material is usually unnecessary."

When the psychiatrist is asked to examine an individual for security purposes or for other legal purposes, such as child custody or to determine job suitability or legal competence, it is incumbent on the psychiatrist to "fully describe the nature and purpose and lack of confidentiality of the examination to the examinee at the beginning of the examination" (*Principles*, Section 4, Annotation 6). The psychiatrist should also define what choices, if any, the interviewee has to accept or refuse to cooperate with such an evaluation.

Psychiatrists are sometimes asked to treat a minor. Section 4, Annotation 7 of the *Principles* states that "careful judgment must be exercised by the psychiatrist in order to include, when appropriate, the parents or guardian in the treatment of a minor. At the same time, the psychiatrist must assure the minor proper confidentiality." Precisely what age defines "minor" in what context varies from state to state and thus requires some knowledge of local laws. Ensuring confidentiality to minors may be relatively easy clinically with young children but difficult—and important—for many teenage patients. Chapter 2 of this primer discusses this issue further.

Section 4, Annotation 8 of the *Principles* states that "psychiatrists at times may find it necessary, in order to protect the patient or the community from imminent danger, to reveal confidential information disclosed by the patient." The area of dangerousness is in part, but not fully, covered by laws and judicial decisions in many states (e.g., *Tarasoff*, *Garamella v. New York Medical College*, *Thapar v. Zezulka*). These have been changing in recent years. An ethical psychiatrist should be familiar with the relevant local laws, precedents, and clinical traditions about duties to warn; should know that ethical dilemmas in this area persist; and should often ask for consultation if the question of major imminent dangerousness arises.

At times the psychiatrist is ordered by a court to reveal information about a patient. Section 4, Annotation 9 of the *Principles* takes up this issue: "When the psychiatrist is ordered by the court to reveal the confidences entrusted to him/her by patients, he/she may comply or he/she may ethically hold the right to dissent within the framework of the law. When the psychiatrist is in doubt, the right of the patient to confidentiality and, by extension, to unimpaired treatment should be given priority. The psychiatrist should reserve the right to raise the question of adequate need for disclosure. In the event that the necessity for legal disclosure is demonstrated by the court, the psychiatrist may request the right to disclosure of only that information which is relevant to the legal question at hand" (*Principles*). Young psychiatrists often do not know that a subpoena is less compelling than a court order and should ensure that they obtain legal consultation as a precaution or when faced with such issues. Furthermore, the ethical psychiatrist should anticipate, and consider in advance with the patient, some instances in which a court might at some point wish to intrude, as in the psychotherapy of a parent in a custody dispute.

Confidentiality issues related to treating severely mentally ill patients somewhat parallel the confidentiality issues related to treating children. The severely mentally ill include those who at least sometimes have significantly impaired judgment (e.g., patients with psychosis, mania, severe depression, delusions, or dementia; or who show signs of dangerousness or acute drug impairment). With these patients, thoughtful involvement of family and/or friends, institutions, or other caregivers may be an important part of good treatment. Deciding to disclose confidential information may be difficult; but, even here, some considered rationing of shared psychiatric material is usually ethically necessary. Psychiatrists frequently have questions about confidentiality in treating the severely mentally ill and are usually aided by consultation and supervision.

Managed care and insurance companies have created many ethical dilemmas for psychiatrists (see Chapter 5 of this primer). Business ethics, such as they are, often clash with medical ethics. Several components of the American Psychiatric Association, including the Ethics

Committee, have tried and are continuing to try, without great success, to define some adequately strong principles that counterbalance managed care and its often sweeping demands for patient information. Time-limited and narrowly defined releases for information are of some, but limited, help. Often driven by short-term profit thinking and not benefiting the patient in question, such demands often overpower psychiatric ethics or wear out doctors and patients—or both—to meet the goal of less payment for care. Facing the economic power of managed care and insurance companies, doctors repeatedly have to weigh the ethical protection of confidentiality against the risk that an insurer will not pay—or will pay very little without long paperwork arguments—and that a particular patient may not get care if his or her insurance company does not pay. This clash of business practice with medical treatment is an area that clearly demands further ethical work, for the health and protection of patients and the psychiatric profession. Some of the work will probably have to occur at a government and legal level.

The relationship of military psychiatry and confidentiality also remains, to many psychiatrists, an area that needs continuing review.

Some additional areas of special confidentiality pitfalls include couples therapy, family therapy, and group therapy. Some customs about confidentiality have evolved in these three areas, and forethought about confidentiality specific to these modalities will help reduce potential confidentiality problems.

Finally, in this incomplete list of potential confidentiality problem areas, comes death. Confidentiality of psychiatric information about patients remains ethically in force after the death of the patient and after the death of the psychiatrist. With only a few exceptions (e.g., those involving court orders, heirs, or executors) and despite the wishes of biographers and historians, it is important for the protection of past, present, and future patients that confidentiality does not end with their or the psychiatrist's death.

Conclusion

Let us return to our original fundamental theme: keep patient material fully confidential at all times unless there is a very strong ethical reason not to do so. And if, in a specific instance, you think there is a reason not to do so, be careful and thoughtful about any exception to patient confidentiality you are tempted to make—and read about such ethical issues, get consultation for the issues encountered, or both.

⌒

References

American Psychiatric Association: The Principles of Medical Ethics With Annotations Especially Applicable to Psychiatry. Washington, DC, American Psychiatric Association, 2001

American Psychiatric Association Committee on Confidentiality: Guidelines on confidentiality. Am J Psychiatry 144:1522–1526, 1987

7

Gifts

Daniel S. Polster, M.D.

In this chapter, we will discuss the ethics of accepting gifts both from patients and from the pharmaceutical or other industry. Although the ethics of accepting gifts from industry may be similar in psychiatry as in other fields of medicine, accepting gifts from patients may be much more complicated. Therefore, the latter topic will be discussed first and in greater detail.

Gifts From Patients

Psychiatrists may occasionally be challenged when patients or their families attempt to give them gifts. This issue is not as black and white as that of sexual boundary violations, and often the appropriate action in dealing with patients' gifts must be evaluated on a case-by-case basis. The decision of whether or not accepting a gift from a patient is ethical may be affected by several factors, including the nature and cost of the gift, the therapeutic relationship between the doctor and patient, and the transference issues that lead to giving the gift. One particular clinical vignette from our residency program illustrates this point rather well.

> A male fourth-year resident at a university hospital began seeing a male undergraduate who was suffering from major depression. The resident saw the patient for three to four sessions for medication management, and the patient improved significantly with a standard dose

of a selective serotonin reuptake inhibitor. The patient and his family were quite grateful for the dramatic improvement and wanted to thank the resident. They were of Middle Eastern descent and felt it appropriate in their culture to purchase a small gift for someone who had helped them so much. At the fourth appointment, the patient brought the resident a gift of a small lamp to be put in his office. The resident, not having faced this situation before, accepted the gift with some hesitation and later presented the case to his two supervisors, a psychopharmacologist in a large, university-based practice and an analyst with a private practice. The analytic supervisor insisted that the resident "return the gift immediately." The psychopharmacologist gave him the opposite advice: "Returning that gift will alienate the patient and his family. Do not return it." The resident decided to keep the gift, the relationship with the patient did not seem affected, and the patient went on to a full recovery.

Why the difference of opinion? Was one of these physicians being unethical, or was each of them speaking from a different personal experience? Is accepting a gift from a patient sometimes ethical? The answer to the last question, made with some hesitation, is "Yes."

Clearly, this issue cannot be served by a blanket statement that accepting gifts is either always or never acceptable. The issue must be addressed in each individual case by asking and answering a few questions: Will the acceptance or refusal of a gift adversely affect the health and well-being of a patient? What is the meaning behind the gift?

It is unethical for psychiatrists to encourage their patients to give them gifts. This likely does not happen often. Yet, patients may give gifts for a multitude of reasons: they are grateful for the care given them, it is the holiday season, or perhaps the gift is just "an innocent gesture of goodwill" (Lyckhom 1998). When the reason behind the gift appears truly benign, accepting it may be ethical. In such cases, not accepting the gift may cause a patient to feel rejected and unwanted, feelings that may be significantly countertherapeutic.

In these cases, considering the cost and nature of the gift is also important. Most small gifts are likely ethical to accept. However, putting a dollar figure on what constitutes a "small gift" is difficult. For one patient, a $10 box of chocolates may be pocket change, whereas for another, that amount may be his or her daily food money. When the gift represents a significant financial burden to the patient, accepting the gift is likely unethical. The situation becomes much more complicated if one is treating a wealthy patient who purchases an expensive gift, yet does not consider it expensive given his or her financial standing. Although one does not want that same patient to feel rejected, the psychiatrist must recognize whether the patient has an unconscious motivation to give the gift and whether the physician's acceptance is based in part on his or her own personal gratification. Acceptance of large or extravagant gifts by the psychiatrist may represent a "serious boundary transgression" (Gabbard and Nadelson 1995). A large financial donation to an institution by a wealthy patient might be publicly acknowledged, but giving that patient special consideration or attention because of the gift is unethical. Especially large or expensive gifts should be acknowledged publicly, then directed to an appropriate charity or foundation (Lyckhom 1998).

The nature of the gift itself must also be considered. Accepting an extremely intimate gift such as lingerie would be unethical, as would gifts of money for the physician's personal use. In such cases, we begin to suspect that a patient's motivation for giving a gift is not so innocent. Giving the gift may represent an attempt to equalize the power structure of the relationship or to seduce the physician, or may be a conscious or unconscious bribe (Lyckhom 1998). It is important that the treating psychiatrist be aware of transference issues present in the therapy as a possible basis for the patient's gift. In some instances, accepting a gift could perpetuate an erotic or other transference and could be quite harmful to the therapeutic relationship—and ultimately to the patient. Accepting gifts in such instances is unethical.

The setting and nature of the therapeutic relationship come into play here as well, such that accepting certain gifts from a patient seen yearly for a medication check might be permissible, whereas accepting the same gifts from a patient in analysis would not be. In the vignette described earlier, the difference in opinion between the two supervising psychiatrists may have its basis in ethics as well as clinical judgment. From the analyst's experience, accepting gifts from patients is unethical and clinically unsound because it clouds the therapeutic relationship and transgresses boundaries. From the pharmacologist's perspective, the patient is being managed with medications, and more harm would be caused by refusing the gift. Neither is right or wrong, but this example demonstrates the need to look at each case individually and to consider the number of variables at work when a patient gives a gift.

Ultimately, "the best interest of the patient is a fundamental parameter by which to measure whether an action is ethically acceptable" (Lyckhom 1998, p. 1945).

⟍⟋

Gifts From Industry

Most physicians find themselves exposed to pharmaceutical company representatives from the first day of their residencies. Often, the overworked and underpaid resident looks forward to "free" textbooks, food, and other gifts that these drug companies can provide. The question of whether accepting these is ethical has been one of considerable debate. Some physicians clearly take advantage of every social event sponsored by the pharmaceutical industry, whereas others refuse even to speak with the representatives who stop by their offices. This issue is faced not only by psychiatrists but by other physicians as well. Are there ethical standards to go by?

The American Medical Association (AMA) already has opinions on gifts to physicians from industry. In summary, opinion 8.061 of the AMA Code of Medical Ethics (American Medical Association Council on Ethical and Judicial Affairs 2000–2001) notes—

> Gifts to physicians should benefit patients, relate to the physician's work, and be of minimal value. Drug samples are allowed, but nonretired physicians may not request samples for personal use. Cash gifts are unacceptable. Gifts should not directly help defray costs of attending a continuing medical education activity or compensate a doctor for time spent at the event, with the exception of faculty speakers. Continuing medical education activities should be chosen for their educational value only. Gifts should serve a genuine educational purpose. Gifts should not be accepted if strings are attached. Scholarships for medical students or residents to attend educational conferences may be awarded to academic institutions, not individuals.

Clearly, any sort of direct reimbursement for prescribing a medication is unethical (Chren et al 1989). However, most situations are less obvious: drug companies may provide physicians with meals, household items, tickets to entertainment, or gifts related to education (e.g., textbooks, journals).

Some feel strongly that such gift giving is unethical in that "inherent in the relationship is an obligation to respond to the gift [which] may influence the physician's decisions with regard to patient care or possibly even erode the physician's character" (Chren et al 1989, p. 3449). The same physicians may feel that gifts from drug companies represent the spending of the patients' money, which is "spent without the patients' knowledge or consent" (Chren et al 1989, p. 3449). They also feel that acceptance of such gifts alters society's perceptions of the profession and establishes some obligation on the part of the physician toward the pharmaceutical company. Ideally, in the minds of the industry, that obligation is to prescribe their medication. Others disagree, stating that such gifts "only facilitate the drug companies' getting enough attention for their products for them to be fairly considered as treatment options and should not be considered unethical" (Gorski 1990).

The inherent obligation may be minimized when gifts are institutional rather than personal. Therefore, it is likely ethical for drug companies to give money to institutions for educational activities, books, or journals in "exchange for only an explicit acknowledgement" (Chren et al 1989). Others feel that gifts such as textbooks or stethoscopes might be unethical as well, since they provide some obligation between the individual and the drug company (Gelbart 1990).

Despite some differences in opinion, the reality is that we live and practice in a world where contact with the pharmaceutical industry is difficult to avoid. Accepting gifts from industry is likely ethical if they contribute to physicians' education or care of patients and do not exceed the norms of pharmaceutical-supported gifts to physicians. Unusually large or extravagant gifts that support neither the physician's education nor patient care likely serve only to increase the physician's obligation to the drug company and are likely unethical. At the same time, one should view gifts presented in the name of education or patient advocacy with some skepticism, keeping in mind that using a company's product solely because of gifts given, rather than using the product because it serves the best interests of the patient, would be unethical.

〜〜

Conclusions

The psychiatrist may be on the receiving end of gifts from both patients and industry throughout his or her career. Although in some instances accepting such gifts may be blatantly unethical, for the most part the issue is less clear and needs to be evaluated on a case-by-case basis. Clinicians can often decide whether accepting gifts is ethical or unethical by asking themselves if doing so—or not doing so—will be in the best interests of their patients.

References

American Medical Association Council on Ethical and Judicial Affairs: Code of Medical Ethics, Current Opinions With Annotations 2000–2001. Chicago, IL, American Medical Association, 2000

Chren MM, Landefeld CS, Murray TH: Doctors, drug companies, and gifts. JAMA 262:3448–3451, 1989

Gabbard GO, Nadelson C: Professional boundaries in the physician–patient relationship. JAMA 273:1445–1449, 1995

Gelbart H: Doctors, drug companies, and gifts (letter). JAMA 263:2177, 1990

Gorski TN: Doctors, drug companies, and gifts (letter). JAMA 263:2177, 1990

Lyckhom LJ: Should physicians accept gifts from patients? JAMA 280:1944–1946, 1998

8

Duty to Report Colleagues Who Engage in Fraud or Deception

Mary Marshall Overstreet, M.D., J.D.

Most of this primer focuses on dealing with potentially unethical behavior, serving as a guide for the many ways in which you may interact with patients. What should you do, however, if concern is raised about the behavior of another psychiatrist?

First, you must be familiar with any legal mandates regarding observations of other physicians. Most states have statutes that require physicians to report observed or even suspected impairment in other physicians to the licensing board for evaluation. Statutes vary widely—most emphasize impairment (e.g., substance abuse or mental or physical illness that affects the ability to practice), but others are broader in terms of poor practice standards or even serious boundary violations, such as sex with patients.

Cases of physician impairment often must be reported to a special committee of the licensing board focused on assessment and rehabilitation, when possible, or on punitive action. Again, statutes vary, but in some states, you may be able to make anonymous reports of such concerns.

Regardless of local law, you also have ethical responsibilities. Principle 2 of *The Principles of Medical Ethics With Annotations Especially Applicable to Psychiatry* (American Psychiatric Association 2001) states in part, "A physician shall...strive to expose those physicians deficient in character or competence, or who engage in fraud or deception." This goes beyond the usual responsibility established in law.

Laws and licensing boards generally focus on issues of public safety; ethics codes and committees set forth and attempt to maintain the highest standards of the profession. These standards tend to be less absolute and more graded than laws or board regulations, requiring more assessment and thoughtful case-by-case evaluation, as illustrated by the other chapters in this primer.

The idea of "reporting" is often uncomfortable, and, in some cultures and countries, reporting other colleagues is not acceptable at all. Every physician has had some experience with adverse outcomes, even in situations of the best informed and most carefully considered and provided treatment. Medicine remains art as well as science and is filled with anxiety-provoking uncertainty. The variables that affect patient well-being are much more numerous than the treatment offered by the physician; yet the recent climate in the United States for litigation or other action often seems not to recognize such facts. These considerations and others, such as a lack of status relative to a supervisor or a more experienced or renowned colleague, can all impede the physician in following the ethical mandate to intervene when there are concerns.

It is important to remember that professions hold special knowledge not usually shared or understood by those outside the profession. Not only is special knowledge part of the profession, but the way the knowledge is used in practice is also part of the standards or unique understanding of the profession's members. Because the standards come from within, it is the members of that profession who are best positioned to establish and maintain or enforce them—a responsibility for significant self-regulation. Thus, the responsibility for self-regulation goes beyond the professional regulations of initial licensing, periodic recredentialing, or specialty certification. With the proliferation of medical advances, many of these regulatory processes are more focused on information than on the manner in which the information is applied or used. Without day-to-day, colleague-to-colleague, and self-to-self attentiveness to aspects of practice broader than specific bits of knowledge, medicine approaches becoming more of a trade than a profession, and the quality of patient care can decline. When an unethical physician continues to practice, this not only harms the patient or patients, but damages the profession as a whole and all potential future patients, who may be reluctant to seek care.

So what does "reporting" or, in the words of Principle 2, "striving to expose" (American Psychiatric Association 2001) mean on a more practical level? The concept is broader than filing a report with a licensing board or ethics committee; "reporting" may in some ways be a misleading shorthand for the variety of responses to a situation of concern. Reporting should encompass actions from a private discussion with a colleague; to clinically appropriate work with a patient who expresses issues arising from prior treatment; to referral of a concern to a departmental committee, a supervisor, or the local American Psychiatric Association (APA) ethics committee for processing. Again, when there are legal mandates, they must also be followed.

Information that creates concern may come from many sources— personal observation or other direct knowledge, media reports, published reports of licensing boards, or statements of patients or even other professionals. Each of these would suggest different initial responses. For example, if you are directly aware that a fellow psychiatrist is having an affair with a patient or former patient, this should be reported to the local APA ethics committee. In many states, such behavior is now also, by statute, criminal and may trigger mandatory reporting to the licensing board. Publications of board findings create an obligation, usually within the local APA leadership, to determine whether a violation of ethical standards occurred. Media information cannot be presumed accurate, but if it is of concern, it should generate some action for further evaluation of the reported conduct. Expressions of concern by other professionals might initially result in a discussion of standards to help them decide whether to pursue some action of their own. (In terms of APA procedures or licensing board investigations, anyone may be a complainant. *The Principles of Medical Ethics With Annotations Especially Applicable to Psychiatry* includes a section that describes the APA's procedures for handling complaints of members' unethical conduct.)

Your own knowledge of consistent, troubling reports over time might be more likely to generate an obligation to speak with the colleague in question or to otherwise attempt to acquire more, or more direct, information. Statements by patients, especially about prior treatment relationships, are often the most difficult to evaluate and require strong clinical skills in assessing the likely accuracy of the information, the potential contribution of past or present psychopathology, and the not-infrequent request that you "not tell anybody about what happened." Obtaining further information or taking action may be limited by constraints of the patient's right to confidentiality.

Whereas the APA Code of Ethics establishes duties to patients, to society, and to better the profession, when these duties conflict, they should always be resolved in favor of the patient. If appropriate, clinical work with the patient may include helping the patient recognize options for his or her own action and may help the patient reach a decision regarding this. Similarly, information gained about a physician in a confidential relationship with him or her should not be shared unless an apparent severe risk exists for the public or other members of the profession, generally cases in which there would be a legal mandate to report.

Issues of physician competency, although generating ethical concerns, should not be determined by any individual, but by an appropriate peer review board. In addition, in carrying out your obligation to assist in maintaining the highest professional standards, you should keep in mind the additional ethical mandates in *The Principles of Medical Ethics With Annotations Especially Applicable to Psychiatry:* "deal honestly with…colleagues" (Principle 2) and "respect the rights…of colleagues" (Principle 4) (American Psychiatric Association 2001).

Some cases of ethical violations will be clear, with a personal observation of another physician's impairment or egregious exploitation; however, in any case of concern, some systematic analysis may be helpful. The following suggestions are proposed to help work through any instance of concern over another psychiatrist's practice or behavior.

First, know your state's laws and licensing board's regulations as well as resources. Failure to follow mandated reporting requirements can result in penalties against you. Resources such as impaired physicians' committees can assess and help a colleague to return to good practice rather than being punitive or letting impairment go unaddressed until something quite serious occurs.

Second, whenever concerns arise, develop and understand them. Consider factors such as why the concern is occurring, evaluate the source of the information, attempt to increase or confirm the information, determine what sort of violation of standards might be involved, and be attentive to any personal values or emotions aroused by the information. For example, are there reasons you are extremely reluctant to address the situation; are your concerns related more to differences with the colleague in style, culture, or treatment orientation than to clear issues of ethical practice?

Third, attempt to identify all potential options for action: discussion with the physician in question; consultation with other colleagues while maintaining the anonymity of the one about whom you are concerned; reports of concern to those in a supervisory role such as a clinical supervisor, residency director, or department head; clinical interventions with a patient; or actual reports of concern to ethics committees, licensing boards, or other peer review bodies. Identify the competing interests inherent in each option and, again, identify personal reactions to each potential option and the impact these may have on the decision-making process.

Fourth, choose an initial option, recognizing that you have identified still other alternatives. Recognize that the goals are maintaining the highest standards of the profession and sustaining trustworthiness to current and all potential future patients.

Reference

American Psychiatric Association: The Principles of Medical Ethics With Annotations Especially Applicable to Psychiatry. Washington, DC, American Psychiatric Association, 2001

9

Ethics of Emergency Care

Beverly J. Fauman, M.D.

Ethical conflicts are as likely to arise in the course of assessment and decision making in an emergency situation as in any other psychiatric setting. Careful consideration must be given to these decisions, even though they must often be made quickly and with little information, because of the short-term, long-term, and potentially life-threatening consequences.

The psychiatrist must act ethically with the emergency patient as with all patients. However, the following areas, discussed in several sections of *The Principles of Medical Ethics With Annotations Especially Applicable to Psychiatry* (American Psychiatric Association 2001), are particularly susceptible to ethical conflict in the emergency situation (Larkin et al. 1994; Mayer and Thibodeau 1997; McCurdy et al. 1996; Montoya 1994; Young et al. 1993).

Section 1

A physician shall be dedicated to providing competent medical service with compassion and respect for human dignity.

Compassion and respect for human dignity are more difficult to sustain in dealing with some chronically mentally ill patients, whose appearance or methods of communication may cause the physician to respond as though the patient were retarded or immature. This was illustrated by the experience of a patient well known to the community mental health center associated with a major university.

> The patient arrived in the waiting room of the community mental health clinic, oozing serosanguinous fluid from between his fingers, which were pressed to his chest. The staff, thinking he had just been assaulted, encouraged the patient to go to an emergency department because the clinic was not equipped to handle the medical problem he appeared to have. He refused to leave, saying he was afraid of the emergency department. Finally, a psychiatrist he knew began to question him as to his obvious physical signs and determined that recent surgery, not an acute injury, was producing the effluence. Arrangements were made to have him seen in the surgery clinic. The patient related that whenever he went to an emergency department, the staff generally did not inquire about physical illness because he was so obviously psychiatrically chronically ill. He observed that only the mental health center staff listened to him.

Psychiatric patients who come to an emergency department even with obvious physical illness often are sent directly to the psychiatrist, frequently without even a determination of vital signs. This is sometimes due to the behavior of the patient, who either does not want to speak to anyone other than a psychiatrist or who acts in a bizarre or psychotic manner. The patient may attribute his or her physical symptoms to delusional causes.

> A 78-year-old man was sent to the emergency department from his senior citizens' housing unit because he was being disruptive repeatedly at night. He volunteered that he had to stay up all night to keep the witches from coming into his window; furthermore, he felt that banging on the windows was additional insurance that they would stay away. Careful questioning revealed that he had decided they came in at night whenever he fell asleep, because when he woke up on those mornings, his legs were swollen. Treatment with haloperidol and digitalis enabled him to return to his home.

Psychiatric patients often anticipate being misunderstood or mistreated in general medical settings. Often, the emergency physician may collude with the psychiatric patient in this regard, since such patients can make other physicians anxious and eager to refer the patient to psychiatry. For example, acutely paranoid patients may respond with hostility to a request to remove their clothes or bare their arms so that blood pressure or pulse can be checked.

A woman presented to the emergency department demanding an examination to confirm her belief that she had been raped the night before. As she further described the assault, the emergency physician concluded that the patient was delusional, since she stated that she had been asleep throughout the attack and nothing in her apartment was disturbed. He decided to request a psychiatric consultation immediately, but she refused and demanded to leave the hospital. He barred her way, insisting on the consultation, at which point she began to threaten him. He then felt he had grounds to commit her and became even more forceful in restricting her departure. By the time the psychiatrist arrived, the tension in the examining room was extreme. The psychiatrist resolved the immediate impasse by ascertaining that the patient's threat was only in response to the provocation she felt and that she was not in any immediate danger to herself or anyone else. He allowed her to leave.

Maintaining a sense of respect or human compassion for patients who are psychotic, threatening, or manic may be difficult, but remembering that the patient still has the right to refuse treatment recommendations is essential, until a decision has been made to commit the patient to some sort of confinement. Even when confined, patients have the right to refuse medication unless their lives are at immediate risk or unless they will likely endanger others' lives. Furthermore, patients have the right to refuse medical treatment, such as chemotherapy for a malignancy, even when their reasons for doing so are based on delusional beliefs.

Patients with no underlying psychiatric disorder may present with behavioral symptoms that are caused by a medical illness. Here, also, patients are frequently referred to a psychiatrist before their illnesses have been adequately assessed. Unfortunately, psychiatric diagnoses tend to stay with patients even when the true etiology is later identified. This can affect a patient's ability to obtain insurance, employment, further medical care, or a security clearance. Custody of minor children may be influenced by a diagnosis of a major psychiatric illness. Even though laws now protect the rights of patients with psychiatric illness, these laws are often breached surreptitiously, for example, by employers. Consider carefully any psychiatric diagnosis applied to a patient for the first time. Whenever some uncertainty exists, less stigmatizing options, such as acute stress reaction or adjustment disorder, give patients the benefit of the doubt.

A patient presented to the emergency department with a description of such bizarre symptoms that she was fairly quickly admitted to the psychiatric unit without undergoing much more than a cursory evaluation in the emergency department. On the psychiatric unit, during the physical examination, the combination of markedly depressed vital signs, "hung-up" reflexes, and a 12-inch well-healed scar at the base of her throat led to the diagnosis of hypothyroid disorder, secondary to the removal of her thyroid gland some 20 years earlier. Laboratory studies and rapid response to thyroid replacement confirmed the diagnosis. The patient did not quite understand the ramifications of her condition and had stopped taking the thyroid medication soon after discharge, because she felt well. When she was brought back to the emergency department approximately 3 months later, treatment of her myxedema coma was delayed because the emergency department staff remembered that she had been admitted to the psychiatric unit on her previous visit and presumed she was now catatonic.

In an emergency, clinicians often do not have all the information needed to make a diagnosis. Psychiatric diagnosis, however, is not the most important task of an emergency assessment. The first obligation is to preserve life, stabilize the patient, assess the circumstances surrounding the situation, and determine the best next step. Diagnoses such as schizophrenia and bipolar disorder cannot be made with certainty with a single episode of illness. Major depressive disorder also implies that the patient's symptoms have been present for a period of time, and although the patient may give a fairly convincing history to support the diagnosis, often there is insufficient evidence to be certain.

Other issues that relate to Section 1 of *The Principles of Medical Ethics* include certifying a patient for treatment, maintaining confidentiality, and being honest with patients. These issues are discussed in more detail in other chapters of this primer.

Section 2

A physician shall deal honestly with patients and colleagues.

Dealing with a patient honestly in an emergency situation becomes conflictual when a psychiatrist determines the need to hospitalize a patient and the patient refuses to sign in. Common practice in this instance involves marshaling resources, such as security guards, other health care personnel, and transportation—as well as contacting the receiving hospital—before alerting the patient of an intention to certify him or her; this is done out of concern that the patient would try to leave the emergency department if he or she knew about the hospitalization. Reassuring a patient falsely until one has control of the situation is not unusual.

Certification deprives the patient of significant personal freedoms and may in the future harm him or her if used by another to obtain certain legal advantages against the patient (e.g., custody of minor children, leverage in a divorce action, power of attorney). The patient may be stigmatized by a history of psychiatric hospitalization, when, in fact, the patient's signs and symptoms were caused by an organic illness that was misdiagnosed. Furthermore, certification may not necessarily accomplish the objective of getting treatment for the patient, even when the etiology is psychiatric. History of a psychiatric hospitalization stigmatizes a patient not only by the implied impairment that occasioned the hospitalization, but also by the blow to one's self-esteem from the experience. Even when a patient agrees to sign into a hospital voluntarily, the agreement may be coerced by a threat of commitment. Unlike rules regarding informed consent, it is not only difficult to identify the risks and benefits of psychiatric hospitalization, but it is also uncertain whether the acutely ill psychiatric patient is able to comprehend them.

In situations of domestic violence or child abuse, a clinician may forgo his or her obligation to be honest with the patient. The staff may deceive the parent or spouse to gain time while arranging for a judicial order or transportation to emergency shelter. When a patient is the child or the battered spouse and his or her safety is the primary concern, no conflict exists. When the assailant is the patient, an ethical dilemma arises that may not be resolved in the short term.

Section 3

A physician shall respect the law and also recognize a responsibility to seek changes in those requirements which are contrary to the best interests of the patient.

Laws regarding commitment vary from state to state and have undergone significant changes over the last couple of decades. Nonetheless, psychiatrists often feel bound by the legal constraints of certification petitions. These address the need for society's protection from a patient but may not permit the psychiatrist to treat the patient, only to contain him or her.

Honesty is also one of the guiding ethical principles in this section, and conflicts arise in the discovery of illegal behavior, such as child abuse or abuse of illicit substances; the former mandates a duty to report the patient, which may substantially interfere with the psychiatrist's ability to encourage the patient to get into treatment. The patient must be informed that legal obligations of the psychiatrist necessitate reporting, commitment, and limits to confidentiality. Some states have so-called "Miranda" rules, which declare that the patient must be informed ahead of time that statements he or she may make to the psychiatrist, such as expressed threats of harm to others or of suicidal intent, may be used to justify an involuntary hospitalization. Mandatory reporting of child abuse or elder abuse overrides the promise to a patient, whether explicit or implied, to maintain confidentiality.

At times, a second psychiatrist may be necessary to evaluate the patient and complete the certification paperwork, when the first psychiatrist has begun an assessment before recognizing that the patient may need to be hospitalized. An ethical dilemma may arise under these circumstances if the patient subsequently denies thoughts or acts that were revealed to the first psychiatrist. Alternatively, when the psychiatrist promises confidentiality, he or she could explain that exclusions exist according to the constraints of the law. This unfortunately may cause the patient to be quite guarded in the information he or she supplies.

⌒⌒

Section 4

A physician shall safeguard
patient confidences within the
constraints of the law.

Some of the problems that present in the emergency situation have been discussed in prior sections of this chapter. Confidentiality may also be unintentionally violated in the emergency situation. The psychiatrist must consider whether he or she actually has the right to examine the patient. A patient who has come to an emergency department for treatment of a self-inflicted injury, treatment of an unexpected reaction to a drug or medication, or treatment of injuries sustained in domestic violence may not want to talk to a psychiatrist. Yet the patient's disclosures to the initial treating physician may directly result in the physician's request for a psychiatric consultation. Family members who express concern about the patient want reassuring information, which the psychiatrist may not be at liberty to reveal.

> A 21-year-old student had a psychotic episode while attending college several hundred miles from his home. Although his parents were aware that his phone calls to them over the previous few weeks had seemed increasingly disjointed and even bizarre, they did not appreciate the degree of looseness of thought and associations that was observed in the emergency department. The patient did not want his parents to be notified, fearing that they would pull him out of school. When the family contacted the treating psychiatrist, she was obliged to explain that no information about the patient could be divulged.

This decision may not appear to be in the patient's best interests. Remember, however, that the family does have other resources, such as the patient himself, the roommate, or possibly the dean of the college. Maintaining confidentiality in such a circumstance is uncomfortable but is an ethical imperative. Permission to speak with family members, to obtain additional information that may help assess and treat the patient, may be denied by that patient. Other facilities that have knowledge about the patient appropriately guard the legal right of the patient not to release any information to family and any other non-medical individuals, even when the information may facilitate the patient's assessment and hasten stabilization. This circumstance is quite similar to the health care provider withholding the patient's history of diabetes or cancer from family and non-medical individuals. Health care providers sometimes disclose this information; however, they should apply the same ethical principle of confidentiality to all medical information.

Confidentiality is difficult to protect when approaching an acutely ill psychiatric patient in the company of other staff, which is often necessary. Security guards, aides, or other staff may need to be present when action is required—for example, with the discovery of behavior that is illegal or dangerous to the patient or others.

Section 6

A physician is free to choose whom to serve, with whom to associate, and the environment in which to provide medical services.

The principle of freedom of choice does not extend to the emergency situation. Thus, even when a psychiatrist has not chosen to practice in an emergency setting, emergencies may arise in which the psychiatrist will be obliged to treat patients he or she would ordinarily not wish to treat. Until the care of the patient has been delegated to another, the psychiatrist must continue to treat such a patient until he or she is stabilized and safe to release. The psychiatrist must balance the care of each patient with the care of other patients and must resist the demand to discharge a patient because of pressures exerted by financial concerns, just as assuredly as he or she must attempt to prevent hospitalization through competent crisis management.

References

American Psychiatric Association: The Principles of Medical Ethics With Annotations Especially Applicable to Psychiatry. Washington, DC, American Psychiatric Association, 2001

Larkin GL, Moskop J, Sanders A, Derse A: The emergency physician and patient confidentiality: a review. Ann Emerg Med 24:1161–1167, 1994

Mayer D, Thibodeau L: Ethical issues in alcohol-related emergencies and emergency care of alcoholic and intoxicated patients, in Advances in Bioethics, Vol 3: Values, Ethics, and Alcoholism. Edited by Shelton WN, Edwards RB. Greenwich, CT, JAI Press, pp 287–308, 1997

McCurdy DB, Brown FB, Shackelton RA, et al: Disclosure vs confidentiality when disaster strikes. Making Rounds in Health, Faith, and Ethics. 22:1:1, 3–5, 1996

Montoya MA: If I tell you, will you treat me? John Marshall Law Review 27:363–372, 1994

Young EWD, Corby JC, Johnson R: Does depression invalidate competence? Consultants' ethical, psychiatric, and legal considerations. Camb Q Healthc Ethics 2:505–515, 1993

10

Ethics and
Forensic Psychiatry

Robert M. Wettstein, M.D.

Ethical issues in forensic psychiatry are perhaps more complex than ethics in the practice of general psychiatry. Many professional responsibilities and activities of forensic psychiatry are unique to the field, a subspecialty of psychiatry. Forensic psychiatrists serve as both treating and evaluating clinicians, and the latter role has drawn the most concern from an ethics perspective, given the adversarial context in which such evaluations typically occur.

The American Academy of Psychiatry and the Law (AAPL; 1995) has endorsed the following definition of forensic psychiatry:

> Forensic psychiatry is a subspecialty of psychiatry in which scientific and clinical expertise is applied to legal issues in legal contexts embracing civil, criminal, correctional or legislative matters: forensic psychiatry should be practiced in accordance with guidelines and ethical principles enunciated by the profession of psychiatry.

This chapter briefly reviews some important ethical issues in the practice of forensic psychiatry, including ethical theory, codes of ethics, boundary issues, and management of allegations of ethical misconduct. For further consideration of these topics, please see Rosner 1994; Rosner and Weinstock 1990; Sales and Simon 1993 in the Suggested Reading section at the end of this chapter.

Ethical Theory in
Forensic Psychiatry

Given the interdisciplinary work of forensic psychiatry, questions arise about what principles of ethics should guide forensic psychiatry and what theory of ethics should underlie those principles.

One perspective is that forensic psychiatry is a subspecialty of psychiatry and a branch of medicine. Should forensic psychiatry be held to the same ethics, rules, and principles as general medicine? Should all physicians be held to the same ethics principles? And should all professional activities of physicians be governed by the same norms of conduct?

One common paradigm of ethical practice in medicine is based on particular principles of medical ethics. The principles reflect historical traditions and social conventions in clinical medicine. These principles include patient autonomy (respecting the decision-making capacity of an autonomous person), beneficence (providing benefits to patients), nonmaleficence (avoiding harm to patients), and justice (fairly distributing costs, benefits, and risks to others) (Beauchamp and Childress 1989). When conflicts arise in a given clinical situation because of the simultaneous application of these principles, physicians attempt to balance the principles, or apply other principles or authority, to resolve the conflict.

Even superficial reflection about the application of these principles reveals that different principles apply depending on the physician's role in the situation. Clearly, physicians, including treating psychiatrists, are obligated to act in the best medical interests of their current patients (i.e., beneficence and nonmaleficence). Physician–scientists performing clinical research, however, are not charged with acting in the best medical interests of their research subjects. Otherwise, placebo-controlled, double-blind research studies, which carry some risk to subjects and not necessarily any individual benefit to them, could not be conducted. Rather, clinical researchers are obligated to work toward the best interests of future patients by collecting valid data and obtaining informed consent for research participation.

Similarly, forensic psychiatrists do not act primarily with beneficence when they conduct pretrial evaluations of litigants in criminal or civil justice proceedings. These evaluations do not serve the litigant-evaluee's best medical interests. Furthermore, in many cases, the results of the evaluation may be harmful to the (nonmedical) financial or legal interests of the evaluee. For example, the evaluator's conclusions may not support the evaluee's claim or defense in the litigation (e.g., nonresponsibility for criminal behavior due to mental illness, or emotional injuries resulting from accidental physical trauma). As a result of the forensic evaluation (at least in part), the criminal defendant may be incarcerated and the civil plaintiff may be denied monetary relief. Such forensic evaluations, however, may be seen as advancing the interests of justice, a larger goal that is distinguished from the interests of the particular litigant (Appelbaum 1997). The forensic psychiatrist assists in the resolution of the legal issue or dispute and, it is hoped, increases the likelihood of a valid result of the litigation by providing critical data about the person or situation.

In basing a theory of ethics for forensic psychiatry on the pursuit of justice rather than on therapeutic principles, Appelbaum (1997) noted that forensic psychiatrists must still be governed by general moral principles in society. When serving the interests of justice, forensic psychiatrists must adhere to the general moral rule of telling the truth (both in the subjective case of honesty and in the objective case of stating the limitations of the accuracy of one's opinions and testimony). Another applicable general moral rule is respect for persons, which requires that the forensic evaluator inform the evaluee of the absence of a physician–patient and treatment relationship between them and of the limits of the confidentiality of the data obtained from the evaluee. Appelbaum (1997) indicated that trying to introduce the principles of medical ethics for treatment into a theory of ethics for forensic psychiatry is perilous.

Another ethics paradigm potentially applicable to forensic psychiatry is that of the adversarial legal system in the United States. The ethical practice of law in the United States is predicated on advocacy, even vigorous advocacy, for the interests of the attorney's client, whether a particular person, an organization, or a branch of government. Forensic psychiatry cannot be governed by the ethics of attorneys, however, because this would simply convert forensic psychiatrists into junior attorneys or advocates for the side that retains them, which is unacceptable (Simon and Wettstein 1997).

Codes of Ethics for Forensic Psychiatry

Two influential groups of forensic mental health professionals have published separate and distinct guidelines for the ethical practice of forensic mental health. The AAPL initially adopted its ethics guidelines in 1987 and has periodically revised them (American Academy of Psychiatry and the Law 1995). Opinions of the AAPL Ethics Committee on particular cases have also been published, analogous to the published opinions of the American Psychiatric Association (APA) Ethics Committee. The Specialty Guidelines for Forensic Psychologists (Committee on Ethical Guidelines for Forensic Psychologists 1991) was adopted by Division 41 of the American Psychological Association, the American Psychology-Law Society, and the American Academy of Forensic Psychology.

The AAPL ethics guidelines focus on confidentiality in forensic evaluations, informed consent to forensic evaluations, honesty and striving for objectivity in conducting forensic evaluations, and the qualifications of forensic examiners. Perhaps the most significant AAPL guideline is that forensic examiners should be honest and strive for objectivity in their assessments. The commentary for this guideline notes that given our adversarial system of legal justice, being retained by one side in a civil or criminal matter exposes forensic psychiatrists to the potential for unintended bias and the danger of distortion of their opinions (American Academy of Psychiatry and the Law 1995). Indeed, even the most ethical, experienced, and conscientious forensic examiner is subject to such "unintended bias" through the process of forensic identification with the retaining side or party. For this reason, the AAPL guidelines prohibit contingency fee arrangements with forensic psychiatric evaluators, because such arrangements are likely to introduce bias into the evaluation process and impair objectivity.

The Specialty Guidelines for Forensic Psychologists is a more detailed and longer document than that published by the AAPL. These specialty guidelines amplify but do not contradict the code of ethics for psychologists published by the American Psychological Association (1991). The Specialty Guidelines for Forensic Psychologists offers an "aspirational model of desirable professional practice by psychologists" (Committee on Ethical Guidelines for Forensic Psychologists 1991, p. 656). The guidelines are useful for those psychologists who either regularly or only occasionally provide forensic psychological services.

Boundary Issues in Forensic Psychiatry

Boundary issues in forensic psychiatric practice are common, as they are in general psychiatric practice. Simon and Wettstein (1997) applied well-known boundary guidelines for the practice of general psychiatry to forensic psychiatric consultation and evaluation. They identified 11 categories of boundary guidelines for the practice of forensic psychiatry: 1) maintain examiner objectivity and neutrality; 2) respect examinee autonomy; 3) protect confidentiality of the forensic evaluation; 4) obtain informed consent for the forensic evaluation unless the evaluation is properly compelled by law; 5) interact verbally with the examinee; 6) ensure no previous, current, or future personal relationship with the examinee; 7) avoid sexual contact with the examinee; 8) preserve the relative anonymity of the evaluator; 9) establish a clear, noncontingent fee policy with the retaining party; 10) provide a suitable examination setting for the evaluation; and 11) define the time and length of the evaluation.

One of the most common ethical dilemmas in forensic practice is the boundary confusion between the role of the treating psychiatrist and that of the forensic psychiatrist in a given case. The AAPL indicates in its ethics guidelines that "treating psychiatrists should generally avoid agreeing to be an expert witness or to perform evaluations of their patients for legal purposes because a forensic evaluation usually requires that other people be interviewed and testimony may adversely affect the therapeutic relationship" (American Academy of Psychiatry and the Law 1995, p. 3). Strasburger and colleagues (1997) have articulated the view that "fundamental incompatibilities" exist between the clinical and the forensic-legal functions of a psychotherapist, and that psychiatrists and other psychotherapists should not serve simultaneously as therapist and forensic evaluator. Attempting to serve both functions simultaneously often results in serving neither one adequately, because the psychotherapy can be compromised in the service of the forensic evaluation, and the forensic evaluation can be compromised by the therapeutic component of the relationship with the evaluee-patient (Greenberg and Shuman 1997).

⌒⌒

Enforcement of Ethical Practice in Forensic Psychiatry

Allegations of unethical practice of forensic psychiatry are brought to APA district branch ethics committees, and thus the APA Ethics Committee, on a regular basis. These formal complaints are brought by patients, evaluees, family members, and others and allege a variety of unethical practices. The district branch and APA ethics committees are obligated to apply *The Principles of Medical Ethics With Annotations Especially Applicable to Psychiatry* (American Psychiatric Association 2001) in determining whether an allegation against an APA member constitutes ethical misconduct. Some published opinions of the APA Ethics Committee also deal with the conduct of forensic evaluations (American Psychiatric Association 1995).

Several sections of *The Principles of Medical Ethics With Annotations Especially Applicable to Psychiatry* are relevant to the practice of forensic psychiatry:

> Sections 1 and 2 relate to providing competent medical service and practicing outside the area of the psychiatrist's expertise, respectively. General psychiatrists without the necessary specialized forensic training, experience, and expertise risk violating these sections when they perform specialized forensic evaluations, such as when a psychiatrist without child psychiatry training and experience evaluates children for child custody. Sections 1 and 2 also relate to boundary violations and exploitation of the evaluee by the forensic examiner as discussed earlier. These include having romantic or sexual relationships with current evaluees or accepting contingency fees.
>
> Section 1 relates to serving with compassion and respect for human dignity, which is violated by abusive behavior toward the evaluee by the forensic examiner. Section 2 addresses dealing honesty with patients and colleagues. Examples of actions violating this section include improperly claiming credentials or experience while testifying under oath or stating that interviews were conducted, or that documents were reviewed that, in fact, were not conducted or reviewed. More complex situa-

tions, representing possible violations, include the deliberate withholding or distortion of data: the testifying psychiatrist who substantially shades the truth or neglects to disclose information that is harmful to the forensic opinion rendered or who deliberately fails to even obtain other data in the course of the evaluation, which could be harmful to the forensic opinion rendered.

Section 4 addresses the confidentiality of psychiatric data and the limits of that confidentiality. An ethics violation here includes release of otherwise confidential information obtained through the course of the forensic evaluation beyond that permitted by the consultation or the litigation process. Another violation includes failing to disclose the nonconfidentiality of the forensic evaluation process to the evaluee. Section 4, Annotation 13, specifically prohibits pre-arraignment psychiatric examinations except to provide treatment.

Section 7, Annotation 3, prohibits a psychiatrist from offering a professional opinion without conducting a psychiatric examination, but this proscription does not relate to the psychiatrist who offers forensic opinions or court testimony in the course of forensic work (American Psychiatric Association 1995).

Because the APA has not explicitly incorporated the AAPL ethics guidelines into its own annotations, the APA and its district branches cannot specifically use or cite the ethics guidelines of the AAPL or forensic psychology in adjudicating an allegation of an ethics violation against an APA member, even if the accused is a member of the AAPL. Nevertheless, a state board of medicine could conceivably cite the AAPL ethics guidelines to prosecute a psychiatrist who has violated them.

The AAPL has explicitly decided not to investigate or adjudicate questions of unethical conduct against its members or against nonmembers. Specific complaints of unethical conduct against AAPL members are typically referred to the local district branch of the APA. Complaints can also be referred to the physician's state licensing board or to the psychiatric association of other countries for members outside of the United States. The AAPL, however, will consider general or hypothetical questions regarding ethics in forensic psychiatry and will sometimes issue opinions about such matters. The AAPL will expel or suspend a member if the APA or the American Academy of Child and Adolescent Psychiatry expels or suspends the member on grounds of ethics misconduct.

Conclusions

This brief overview of some ethics issues in forensic psychiatry has only introduced some of the complex matters raised by forensic consultation and evaluation. Many other ethics issues exist in specific areas of forensic psychiatry. For instance, ethics issues related to assessing and treating sexual offenders have gained increasing prevalence and importance; sources listed in the Suggested Reading section at the end of this chapter review these ethical issues. Moreover, psychiatry and forensic psychiatry are in search of the moral or ethical theory and operative rules for forensic activities. Much attention is paid to the problem of honesty and objectivity in forensic work, and justifiably so, although some skeptics have asserted that the "impartial expert" is a myth or fallacy, rather than a desired reality or ideal (Diamond 1973). Also, appreciation is growing for the problem of double agency, with psychotherapists wearing the two hats of therapist and forensic evaluator. Ethical standards of behavior for forensic work will continue to evolve, as they do in therapeutic work with patients.

References

American Academy of Psychiatry and the Law: American Academy of Psychiatry and the Law Ethics Guidelines for the Practice of Forensic Psychiatry. Bloomfield, CT, American Academy of Psychiatry and the Law, 1995

American Psychiatric Association: Opinions of the Ethics Committee on The Principles of Medical Ethics With Annotations Especially Applicable to Psychiatry. Washington, DC, American Psychiatric Association, 1995

American Psychiatric Association: The Principles of Medical Ethics With Annotations Especially Applicable to Psychiatry. Washington, DC, American Psychiatric Association, 2001

American Psychological Association: Ethical principles of psychologists and code of conduct. Am Psychol 47:1597–1611, 1991

Appelbaum PS: A theory of ethics for forensic psychiatry. J Am Acad Psychiatry Law 25:233–247, 1997

Beauchamp T, Childress J: Principles of Biomedical Ethics, 3rd Edition. New York, Oxford University Press, 1989

Committee on Ethical Guidelines for Forensic Psychologists: Specialty guidelines for forensic psychologists. Law Hum Behav 15:655–665, 1991

Diamond B: The psychiatrist as advocate. Journal of Psychiatry and Law 1:7–19, 1973

Greenberg SA, Shuman DA: Irreconcilable conflict between therapeutic and forensic roles. Professional Psychology: Research and Practice 28:50–57, 1997

Simon RI, Wettstein RM: Toward the development of guidelines for the conduct of forensic psychiatric examinations. J Am Acad Psychiatry Law 25:17–30, 1997

Strasburger LH, Gutheil TG, Brodsky A: On wearing two hats: role conflict in serving as both psychotherapist and expert witness. Am J Psychiatry 154:448–456, 1997

Suggested Reading

General Ethical Issues in Forensic Psychiatry

Rosner R (ed): Principles and Practice of Forensic Psychiatry. New York, Chapman & Hall, 1994

Rosner R, Weinstock R (eds): Ethical Practice in Psychiatry and the Law. New York, Plenum, 1990

Sales BD, Simon L (eds): The Ethics of Expert Witnessing (special issue). Ethics and Behavior 3:223–393, 1993

Ethical Issues in Assessing and Treating Sexual Offenders

American Psychiatric Association Task Force on Sexually Dangerous Offenders: Dangerous Sex Offenders: A Task Force Report of the American Psychiatric Association. Washington, DC, American Psychiatric Association, 1999

Predators and Politics: A Symposium on Washington's Sexually Violent Predators Statute. University of Puget Sound Law Review 15:507–987, 1992

Wettstein RM: A psychiatric perspective on Washington's sexually violent predators statute. University of Puget Sound Law Review 15:597–633, 1992

11

Consultations and Second Opinions

Gary S. Weinstein, M.D.

In a general hospital setting, the diagnosis and treatment recommendation for psychiatric illness in a medically ill patient must be timely. This chapter introduces ethical issues related to consultations and second opinions for these and other patients seeking psychiatric care. Along with differentiating the cause of abnormal behavior, it is advisable to communicate treatment recommendations clearly, with simple language and concrete recommendations. Each individual hospital's consultation guidelines must be followed. These guidelines often recommend a psychiatric consultation when a patient exhibits suicidality or severe psychiatric symptoms and is not currently under a psychiatrist's care.

A psychiatrist is a licensed physician who can perform physical examinations with proper training and necessary skills. Another psychiatrist or physician can be called on to perform a physical examination for a consultation or a second opinion if this would improve the care of the patient, or if the treating psychiatrist's physical examination under certain circumstances could be harmful.

In the course of a patient's care, a psychiatrist should obtain a consultation whenever it is medically indicated or if the patient requests it. The patient's representative may request a consultation in cases in which the patient is incompetent or a minor. A consultation may also be indicated when a patient's symptoms cause dysfunction despite ongoing treatment, particularly if the dysfunction is severe.

If the treating psychiatrist is frightened by a patient or feels that no treatment might be useful, a consultation with a colleague could be helpful. If this patient is a minor, the parents should be advised of the clinical situation, and the minor should be properly referred for further care.

The treating psychiatrist who refers a patient for consultation should provide the consulting psychiatrist a case history, along with other pertinent information, and should highlight the specific question about which guidance is sought. The treating psychiatrist should also agree to a request for consultation from the patient or the patient's representative, and even though possible consultants may be suggested, the patient or representative should be given free choice. If the psychiatrist disapproves of the professional qualifications of the consultant or if a difference of opinion cannot be resolved, after suitable notice, the treating psychiatrist may withdraw from the case. If this occurs within an institution or agency, arbitration by a higher authority within that institution or agency should first be attempted to resolve differences.

The treating psychiatrist can recommend that a patient obtain a second opinion whenever it is in the best interests of the patient. The patient should be informed of the reasons for the recommendation, and be told that the treating psychiatrist can assist the patient in choosing a psychiatrist for a second opinion, that the patient is free to choose one of his or her own, and that the patient is also free to obtain a second opinion without the treating psychiatrist's knowledge. The treating psychiatrist should then give the psychiatrist who provides a second opinion (a consultation) both a history of the case and current treatment recommendations regarding management and care.

For the treating psychiatrist, terminating the physician–patient relationship because a patient decides to obtain a second opinion is inappropriate. The treating psychiatrist must ask for a consultation when one is indicated and not impede the consultation because of prior paid arrangements or because of moral views.

When referring a patient for consultation, the treating psychiatrist ensures that the referral is to a recognized member of the psychiatrist's own discipline, competent to carry out the tasks required. If the skill or qualifications of that professional are in doubt, the psychiatrist should not refer a patient to that person.

In a collaborative or a supervisory role, sufficient time must be allotted to ensure that proper care is given. The psychiatrist must not be used as a figurehead, since doing so is contrary to the interests of the patient, and the frequency and amount of time spent in this role should not depend on either prior arrangements or availability but on the true need of the patient. A consulting psychiatrist should clarify his or her role as much as possible before seeing the referred patient.

In a hospital setting, the results of the examination that the consulting psychiatrist should give the referral source include formulation, diagnosis, and pertinent recommendations. In other settings, the consulting psychiatrist should give patients an explanation of his or her opinion, providing patients a clear understanding of the opinion, even if it does not agree with the treating psychiatrist's recommendation. The consulting psychiatrist may discuss an opinion with the treating psychiatrist but is not obligated to do so if the patient or representative employs the consulting psychiatrist for advice. A report to the treating psychiatrist can be made if the patient or representative gives consent.

If a psychiatrist is asked to give a second opinion and is asked by the patient to also provide needed medical care, assuming responsibility for that patient's care is within the principles of ethics. When asked to provide a second opinion, the psychiatrist may not establish a prior agreement or understanding of refusal to treat the referred patient. Such agreements are not only unethical, but also unlawful. However, after providing a second opinion, the psychiatrist does not necessarily have to treat a referred patient for the following reasons: 1) as part of an arrangement with insurers or other third-party payers; 2) to avoid any perceived conflict of interest; or 3) to avoid loss of objectivity. Patients exercising the right of free choice may also decide not to seek treatment from the doctor who provided a second opinion.

Ethically, a psychiatrist who consults for an organization can provide consultation or treatment to that organization's members unless an agreement prohibiting this has been made. In addition, an organization is not obligated to refer patients to other psychiatrists, but the psychiatrist should inform these patients that they have the right and freedom to choose another psychiatrist in the community. In this circumstance, as in others above, any conflict of interest should be avoided (American Psychiatric Association 2001).

Reference

American Psychiatric Association: The Principles of Medical Ethics With Annotations Especially Applicable to Psychiatry. Washington, DC, American Psychiatric Association, 2001

Appendix

The Principles of Medical Ethics

With Annotations Especially Applicable to Psychiatry
2001 Edition

In 1973, the American Psychiatric Association published the first edition of *The Principles of Medical Ethics With Annotations Especially Applicable to Psychiatry.* Subsequently, revisions were published as the Board of Trustees and the Assembly approved additional annotations. In July of 1980, the American Medical Association approved a new version of the *Principles of Medical Ethics* (the first revision since 1957) and the APA Ethics Committee[1] incorporated many of its annotations into the new *Principles*, which resulted in the 1981 edition and subsequent revisions.

---

[1]The committee included Herbert Klemmer, M.D., Chairperson, Miltiades Zaphiropoulos, M.D., Ewald Busse, M.D., John R. Saunders, M.D., and Robert McDevitt, M.D. J. Brand Brickman, M.D., William P. Camp, M.D., and Robert A. Moore, M.D., served as consultants to the APA Ethics Committee.

⌒

Foreword

ALL PHYSICIANS should practice in accordance with the medical code of ethics set forth in the *Principles of Medical Ethics* of the American Medical Association. An up-to-date expression and elaboration of these statements is found in the Opinions and Reports of the Council on Ethical and Judicial Affairs of the American Medical Association.[2] Psychiatrists are strongly advised to be familiar with these documents.[3]

However, these general guidelines have sometimes been difficult to interpret for psychiatry, so further annotations to the basic principles are offered in this document. While psychiatrists have the same goals as all physicians, there are special ethical problems in psychiatric practice that differ in coloring and degree from ethical problems in other branches of medical practice, even though the basic principles are the same. The annotations are not designed as absolutes and will be revised from time to time so as to be applicable to current practices and problems.

Following are the AMA *Principles of Medical Ethics*, printed in their entirety, and then each principle printed separately along with an annotation especially applicable to psychiatry.

---

[2]*Current Opinions with Annotations of the Council on Ethical and Judicial Affairs*, Chicago, American Medical Association, 2000–2001.

[3]Chapter 8, Section 1 of the Bylaws of the American Psychiatric Association states, "All members of the Association shall be bound by the ethical code of the medical profession, specifically defined in the *Principles of Medical Ethics* of the American Medical Association and in the Association's *Principles of Medical Ethics With Annotations Especially Applicable to Psychiatry*." In interpreting the Bylaws, it is the opinion of the Board of Trustees that inactive status in no way removes a physician member from responsibility to abide by the *Principles of Medical Ethics*.

Principles of Medical Ethics*
American Medical Association

Preamble

The medical profession has long subscribed to a body of ethical statements developed primarily for the benefit of the patient. As a member of this profession, a physician must recognize responsibility not only to patients but also to society, to other health professionals, and to self. The following principles, adopted by the American Medical Association, are not laws but standards of conduct, which define the essentials of honorable behavior for the physician.

Section 1

A physician shall be dedicated to providing competent medical service with compassion and respect for human dignity.

Section 2

A physician shall deal honestly with patients and colleagues, and strive to expose those physicians deficient in character or competence, or who engage in fraud or deception.

Section 3

A physician shall respect the law and also recognize a responsibility to seek changes in those requirements which are contrary to the best interests of the patient.

Section 4

A physician shall respect the rights of patients, of colleagues, and of other health professionals, and shall safeguard patient confidences within the constraints of the law.

---

*The American Medical Association is expected to approve changes to *Principles of Medical Ethics* later in 2001.

Section 5

A physician shall continue to study, apply, and advance scientific knowledge, make relevant information available to patients, colleagues, and the public, obtain consultation, and use the talents of other health professionals when indicated.

Section 6

A physician shall, in the provision of appropriate patient care, except in emergencies, be free to choose whom to serve, with whom to associate, and the environment in which to provide medical services.

Section 7

A physician shall recognize a responsibility to participate in activities contributing to an improved community.

⌐⌒⌐

Principles With Annotations

Following are each of the AMA *Principles of Medical Ethics* printed separately along with annotations especially applicable to psychiatry.

Preamble

The medical profession has long subscribed to a body of ethical statements developed primarily for the benefit of the patient. As a member of this profession, a physician must recognize responsibility not only to patients but also to society, to other health professionals, and to self. The following Principles, adopted by the American Medical Association, are not laws but standards of conduct, which define the essentials of honorable behavior for the physician.[4]

Section 1

A physician shall be dedicated to providing competent medical service with compassion and respect for human dignity.

---

[4] Statements in italics are taken directly from the American Medical Association's *Principles of Medical Ethics*.

1. A psychiatrist shall not gratify his/her own needs by exploiting the patient. The psychiatrist shall be ever vigilant about the impact that his/her conduct has upon the boundaries of the doctor/patient relationship, and thus upon the well being of the patient. These requirements become particularly important because of the essentially private, highly personal, and sometimes intensely emotional nature of the relationship established with the psychiatrist.

2. A psychiatrist should not be a party to any type of policy that excludes, segregates, or demeans the dignity of any patient because of ethnic origin, race, sex, creed, age, socioeconomic status, or sexual orientation.

3. In accord with the requirements of law and accepted medical practice, it is ethical for a physician to submit his/her work to peer review and to the ultimate authority of the medical staff executive body and the hospital administration and its governing body. In case of dispute, the ethical psychiatrist has the following steps available:

a. Seek appeal from the medical staff decision to a joint conference committee, including members of the medical staff executive committee and the executive committee of the governing board. At this appeal, the ethical psychiatrist could request that outside opinions be considered.

b. Appeal to the governing body itself.

c. Appeal to state agencies regulating licensure of hospitals if, in the particular state, they concern themselves with matters of professional competency and quality of care.

d. Attempt to educate colleagues through development of research projects and data and presentations at professional meetings and in professional journals.

e. Seek redress in local courts, perhaps through an enjoining injunction against the governing body.

f. Public education as carried out by an ethical psychiatrist would not utilize appeals based solely upon emotion, but would be presented in a professional way and without any potential exploitation of patients through testimonials.

4. A psychiatrist should not be a participant in a legally authorized execution.

Section 2

A physician shall deal honestly with patients and colleagues, and strive to expose those physicians deficient in character or competence, or who engage in fraud or deception.

1. The requirement that the physician conduct himself/herself with propriety in his/her profession and in all the actions of his/her life is especially important in the case of the psychiatrist because the patient tends to model his/her behavior after that of his/her psychiatrist by identification. Further, the necessary intensity of the treatment relationship may tend to activate sexual and other needs and fantasies on the part of both patient and psychiatrist, while weakening the objectivity necessary for control. Additionally, the inherent inequality in the doctor-patient relationship may lead to exploitation of the patient. Sexual activity with a current or former patient is unethical.

2. The psychiatrist should diligently guard against exploiting information furnished by the patient and should not use the unique position of power afforded him/her by the psychotherapeutic situation to influence the patient in any way not directly relevant to the treatment goals.

3. A psychiatrist who regularly practices outside his/her area of professional competence should be considered unethical. Determination of professional competence should be made by peer review boards or other appropriate bodies.

4. Special consideration should be given to those psychiatrists who, because of mental illness, jeopardize the welfare of their patients and their own reputations and practices. It is ethical, even encouraged, for another psychiatrist to intercede in such situations.

5. Psychiatric services, like all medical services, are dispensed in the context of a contractual arrangement between the patient and the physician. The provisions of the contractual arrangement, which are binding on the physician as well as on the patient, should be explicitly established.

6. It is ethical for the psychiatrist to make a charge for a missed appointment when this falls within the terms of the specific contractual agreement with the patient. Charging for a missed appointment or for one not canceled 24 hours in advance

need not, in itself, be considered unethical if a patient is fully advised that the physician will make such a charge. The practice, however, should be resorted to infrequently and always with the utmost consideration for the patient and his/her circumstances.

7. An arrangement in which a psychiatrist provides supervision or administration to other physicians or nonmedical persons for a percentage of their fees or gross income is not acceptable; this would constitute fee-splitting. In a team of practitioners, or a multidisciplinary team, it is ethical for the psychiatrist to receive income for administration, research, education, or consultation. This should be based upon a mutually agreed upon and set fee or salary, open to renegotiation when a change in the time demand occurs. (See also Section 5, Annotations 2, 3, and 4.)

Section 3

A physician shall respect the law and also recognize a responsibility to seek changes in those requirements which are contrary to the best interests of the patient.

1. It would seem self-evident that a psychiatrist who is a law-breaker might be ethically unsuited to practice his/her profession. When such illegal activities bear directly upon his/her practice, this would obviously be the case. However, in other instances, illegal activities such as those concerning the right to protest social injustices might not bear on either the image of the psychiatrist or the ability of the specific psychiatrist to treat his/her patient ethically and well. While no committee or board could offer prior assurance that any illegal activity would not be considered unethical, it is conceivable that an individual could violate a law without being guilty of professionally unethical behavior. Physicians lose no right of citizenship on entry into the profession of medicine.

2. Where not specifically prohibited by local laws governing medical practice, the practice of acupuncture by a psychiatrist is not unethical per se. The psychiatrist should have professional competence in the use of acupuncture. Or, if he/she is supervising the use of acupuncture by nonmedical individuals, he/she should provide proper medical supervision. (See also Section 5, Annotations 3 and 4.)

Section 4

A physician shall respect the rights of patients, of colleagues, and of other health professionals, and shall safeguard patient confidences within the constraints of the law.

1. Psychiatric records, including even the identification of a person as a patient, must be protected with extreme care. Confidentiality is essential to psychiatric treatment. This is based in part on the special nature of psychiatric therapy as well as on the traditional ethical relationship between physician and patient. Growing concern regarding the civil rights of patients and the possible adverse effects of computerization, duplication equipment, and data banks makes the dissemination of confidential information an increasing hazard. Because of the sensitive and private nature of the information with which the psychiatrist deals, he/she must be circumspect in the information that he/she chooses to disclose to others about a patient. The welfare of the patient must be a continuing consideration.

2. A psychiatrist may release confidential information only with the authorization of the patient or under proper legal compulsion. The continuing duty of the psychiatrist to protect the patient includes fully apprising him/her of the connotations of waiving the privilege of privacy. This may become an issue when the patient is being investigated by a government agency, is applying for a position, or is involved in legal action. The same principles apply to the release of information concerning treatment to medical departments of government agencies, business organizations, labor unions, and insurance companies. Information gained in confidence about patients seen in student health services should not be released without the students' explicit permission.

3. Clinical and other materials used in teaching and writing must be adequately disguised in order to preserve the anonymity of the individuals involved.

4. The ethical responsibility of maintaining confidentiality holds equally for the consultations in which the patient may not have been present and in which the consultee was not a physician. In such instances, the physician consultant should alert the consultee to his/her duty of confidentiality.

5. Ethically the psychiatrist may disclose only that information which is relevant to a given situation. He/she should avoid offering speculation as fact. Sensitive information such as an individual's sexual orientation or fantasy material is usually unnecessary.

6. Psychiatrists are often asked to examine individuals for security purposes, to determine suitability for various jobs, and to determine legal competence. The psychiatrist must fully describe the nature and purpose and lack of confidentiality of the examination to the examinee at the beginning of the examination.

7. Careful judgment must be exercised by the psychiatrist in order to include, when appropriate, the parents or guardian in the treatment of a minor. At the same time, the psychiatrist must assure the minor proper confidentiality.

8. Psychiatrists at times may find it necessary, in order to protect the patient or the community from imminent danger, to reveal confidential information disclosed by the patient.

9. When the psychiatrist is ordered by the court to reveal the confidences entrusted to him/her by patients, he/she may comply or he/she may ethically hold the right to dissent within the framework of the law. When the psychiatrist is in doubt, the right of the patient to confidentiality and, by extension, to unimpaired treatment should be given priority. The psychiatrist should reserve the right to raise the question of adequate need for disclosure. In the event that the necessity for legal disclosure is demonstrated by the court, the psychiatrist may request the right to disclosure of only that information which is relevant to the legal question at hand.

10. With regard for the person's dignity and privacy and with truly informed consent, it is ethical to present a patient to a scientific gathering, if the confidentiality of the presentation is understood and accepted by the audience.

11. It is ethical to present a patient or former patient to a public gathering or to the news media only if the patient is fully informed of enduring loss of confidentiality, is competent, and consents in writing without coercion.

12. When involved in funded research, the ethical psychiatrist will advise human subjects of the funding source, retain his/her freedom to reveal data and results, and follow all appropriate and current guidelines relative to human subject protection.

13. Ethical considerations in medical practice preclude the psychiatric evaluation of any person charged with criminal acts prior to access to, or availability of, legal counsel. The only exception is the rendering of care to the person for the sole purpose of medical treatment.

14. Sexual involvement between a faculty member or supervisor and a trainee or student, in those situations in which an abuse of power can occur, often takes advantage of inequalities in the working relationship and may be unethical because: (a) any treatment of a patient being supervised may be deleteriously affected; (b) it may damage the trust relationship between teacher and student; and (c) teachers are important professional role models for their trainees and affect their trainees' future professional behavior.

Section 5

A physician shall continue to study, apply, and advance scientific knowledge, make relevant information available to patients, colleagues, and the public, obtain consultation, and use the talents of other health professionals when indicated.

1. Psychiatrists are responsible for their own continuing education and should be mindful of the fact that theirs must be a lifetime of learning.

2. In the practice of his/her specialty, the psychiatrist consults, associates, collaborates, or integrates his/her work with that of many professionals, including psychologists, psychometricians, social workers, alcoholism counselors, marriage counselors, public health nurses, etc. Furthermore, the nature of modern psychiatric practice extends his/her contacts to such people as teachers, juvenile and adult probation officers, attorneys, welfare workers, agency volunteers, and neighborhood aides. In referring patients for treatment, counseling, or rehabilitation to any of these practitioners, the psychiatrist should ensure that the allied professional or paraprofessional with whom he/she is dealing is a recognized member of his/her own discipline and is competent to carry out the therapeutic task required. The psychiatrist should have the same attitude toward members of the medical profession to whom he/she refers patients. Whenever he/she has reason to doubt the

training, skill, or ethical qualifications of the allied professional, the psychiatrist should not refer cases to him/her.

3. When the psychiatrist assumes a collaborative or supervisory role with another mental health worker, he/she must expend sufficient time to assure that proper care is given. It is contrary to the interests of the patient and to patient care if he/she allows himself/herself to be used as a figurehead.

4. In relationships between psychiatrists and practicing licensed psychologists, the physician should not delegate to the psychologist or, in fact, to any nonmedical person any matter requiring the exercise of professional medical judgment.

5. The psychiatrist should agree to the request of a patient for consultation or to such a request from the family of an incompetent or minor patient. The psychiatrist may suggest possible consultants, but the patient or family should be given free choice of the consultant. If the psychiatrist disapproves of the professional qualifications of the consultant or if there is a difference of opinion that the primary therapist cannot resolve, he/she may, after suitable notice, withdraw from the case. If this disagreement occurs within an institution or agency framework, the differences should be resolved by the mediation or arbitration of higher professional authority within the institution or agency.

Section 6

A physician shall, in the provision of appropriate patient care, except in emergencies, be free to choose whom to serve, with whom to associate, and the environment in which to provide medical services.

1. Physicians generally agree that the doctor-patient relationship is such a vital factor in effective treatment of the patient that preservation of optimal conditions for development of a sound working relationship between a doctor and his/her patient should take precedence over all other considerations. Professional courtesy may lead to poor psychiatric care for physicians and their families because of embarrassment over the lack of a complete give-and-take contract.

2. An ethical psychiatrist may refuse to provide psychiatric treatment to a person who, in the psychiatrist's opinion, cannot

be diagnosed as having a mental illness amenable to psychiatric treatment.

Section 7

A physician shall recognize a responsibility to participate in activities contributing to an improved community.

1. Psychiatrists should foster the cooperation of those legitimately concerned with the medical, psychological, social, and legal aspects of mental health and illness. Psychiatrists are encouraged to serve society by advising and consulting with the executive, legislative, and judiciary branches of the government. A psychiatrist should clarify whether he/she speaks as an individual or as a representative of an organization. Furthermore, psychiatrists should avoid cloaking their public statements with the authority of the profession (e.g., "Psychiatrists know that...").

2. Psychiatrists may interpret and share with the public their expertise in the various psychosocial issues that may affect mental health and illness. Psychiatrists should always be mindful of their separate roles as dedicated citizens and as experts in psychological medicine.

3. On occasion psychiatrists are asked for an opinion about an individual who is in the light of public attention, or who has disclosed information about himself/herself through public media. In such circumstances, a psychiatrist may share with the public his/her expertise about psychiatric issues in general. However, it is unethical for a psychiatrist to offer a professional opinion unless he/she has conducted an examination and has been granted proper authorization for such a statement.

4. The psychiatrist may permit his/her certification to be used for the involuntary treatment of any person only following his/her personal examination of that person. To do so, he/she must find that the person, because of mental illness, cannot form a judgment as to what is in his/her own best interests and that, without such treatment, substantial impairment is likely to occur to the person or others.

ADDENDUM 1

Guidelines for Ethical Practice in Organized Settings

At its meeting of September 13–14, 1997, the APA Ethics Committee voted to make the "Guidelines for Ethical Practice in Organized Settings," as approved by the Board and the Assembly, an addendum to *The Principles of Medical Ethics With Annotations Especially Applicable to Psychiatry*, to be preceded by introductory historical comments, and cross-referenced to the appropriate annotations, as follows:

> This addendum to the *The Principles of Medical Ethics With Annotations Especially Applicable to Psychiatry* was approved by the Board of Trustees in March 1997, and by the Assembly of District Branches in May 1997. This addendum contains specific guidelines regarding ethical psychiatric practice in organized settings and is intended to clarify existing ethical standards contained in Sections 1–7.

Addendum

Psychiatrists have a long and valued tradition of being essential participants in organizations that deliver health care. Such organizations can enhance medical effectiveness and protect the standards and values of the psychiatric profession by fostering competent, compassionate medical care in a setting in which informed consent and confidentiality are rigorously preserved, conditions essential for the successful treatment of mental illness. However, some organizations may place the psychiatrist in a position where the clinical needs of the patient, the demands of the community and larger society, and even the professional role of the psychiatrist are in conflict with the interests of the organization.

The psychiatrist must consider the consequences of such role conflicts with respect to patients in his or her care, and strive to resolve these conflicts in a manner that is likely to be of greatest benefit to the patient. Whether during treatment or a review process, a psychiatrist shall respect the autonomy, privacy, and dignity of the patient and his or her family.

These guidelines are intended to clarify existing standards. They are intended to promote the interests of the patient, and should not be construed to interfere with the ability of a psychiatrist to practice in an organized setting. The principles and annotations noted in this communication conform to the statement in the preamble to the *Principles of Medical Ethics*. These are not laws but standards of conduct, which define the essentials of honorable behavior for the physician.

1. **Appropriateness of Treatment and Treatment Options**

    a. A psychiatrist shall not withhold information that the patient needs or reasonably could use to make informed treatment decisions, including options for treatment not provided by the psychiatrist. [Section 1, Annotation 1 (APA); Section 2, Annotation 4 (APA)]

    b. A psychiatrist's treatment plan shall be based upon clinical, scientific, or generally accepted standards of treatment. This applies to the treating and the reviewing psychiatrist. [Section 1, Annotation 1 (APA); Section 2 (APA); Section 4 (APA)]

    c. A psychiatrist shall strive to provide beneficial treatment which shall not be limited to minimum criteria of medical necessity. [Section 1, Annotation 1 (APA)]

2. **Financial Arrangements**
    When a psychiatrist is aware of financial incentives or penalties which limit the provision of appropriate treatment for that patient, the psychiatrist shall inform the patient and/or designated guardian. [Section 1, Annotation 1 (APA); Section 2 (APA)]

3. **Review Process**
    A psychiatrist shall not conduct reviews or participate in reviews in a manner likely to demean the dignity of the patient by asking for highly personal material not necessary for the conduct of the review. A reviewing psychiatrist shall strive as hard for a patient he or she reviews as for one he or she treats to prevent the disclosure of sensitive patient material to anyone other than for clear, clinical necessity. [Section 1, Annotations 1 and 2 (APA); Section 4, Annotations 1, 2, 4, and 5 (APA)]

Index

Adolescents. *See also* Children, psychiatric care of
confidentiality with, 16–17
countertransference with, 19
psychotropic medications for, 15, 16
Alienists, 1
Allocation guidelines restricting care and choices, 35
Alternative treatments, managed care and, 33–34, 35
Altruism, 1
American Academy of Psychiatry and the Law (AAPL), 65, 68, 69, 71–72
American Medical Association (AMA), x, 79
on gifts to physicians from industry, 48
managed care guidelines, 35
Opinions and Reports of Council on Ethical and Judicial Affairs of, 80
principles of medical ethics, x, 81–82. *See also Principles of Medical Ethics With Annotations Especially Applicable to Psychiatry, The* (APA)
American Psychiatric Association (APA), ix–xi, 42, 79. *See also Principles of Medical Ethics With*

Annotations Especially Applicable to Psychiatry, The (APA)
Board of Trustees, 3, 36, 91
Code of Ethics, 54
Ethics Committee, xi, 42–43, 79, 91
ethics committees, xi, 53, 55
enforcement in forensic psychiatry by, 70–71, 72
Guidelines for Ethical Practice in Organized Settings, 91–92
guidelines of practice for managed care reviewers, 36–37
Office of Ethics and Professional Responsibility, xi
Appeals of dispute over physician competency, 83
Appropriateness of treatment and treatment options, 92
Aspirin, use on children of, 15
Assent, 12, 15. *See also* Informed consent
Autonomy, patient, 24, 66
opposition to involuntary treatment based on, 28
paternalism vs., 8, 24, 28
use of restraints and decrease in, 26

Barter arrangements, 7–8
Beneficence, principle of, 28, 66

93

Boundary violations, 1–9
  boundary crossings, 2–9
  forensic psychiatry and, 69
  nonsexual, 4–9
    autonomy, 8
    confidentiality, 7
    employing a patient, 7
    financial relationships, 7–8
    gifts, 5–6, 47
    influences, 8–9
    information, 8, 84
    physical contact, 6–7
    self-disclosure, 4–5
  in psychiatric care of children,
    20–21
  sexual, 3–4, 20, 84
  therapeutic frame and its
    boundaries, 1–2, 83
  vigilance to avoid, 83
Business ethics, clash between
  medical ethics and, 42–43. *See
  also* Managed care

California
  confidentiality exceptions with
    child patients, 18
  informed consent for children in
    foster care, 13–14
Capitation fees, 34
Caregiver, self-disclosure and patient
  as, 5
Case presentation, 40, 86, 87
Certification. *See also*
  Hospitalization
  forgoing obligation to be honest
    with patient in cases of, 60–61
  for involuntary treatment, 90
  legal constraints of, 62
  stigma of, 61
Child abuse
  forgoing obligation to be honest
    with patient in cases of, 61
  mandatory reporting of, 17–18, 62

Children, psychiatric care of, 11–22
  boundary violations in, 20–21
  confidentiality in, 16–18, 41, 87
  developmental issues in, 11, 12, 15
  emancipated minors, 13, 14, 18
  in foster care, 13–14
  hospitalization, 21–22
  infants, 11
  informed consent and, 12–14
  medical records of, 18
  psychopharmacology and, 14–16
  psychotherapy with families and
    children, 18–20
Citizen, physician's role as
  dedicated, 90
Clinical researchers, medical ethics
  principles and, 66
Code of Ethics, AMA, 48
Code of Ethics, APA, 54
Codes of ethics for forensic
  psychiatry, 68
Coercion, 24
  involuntary hospitalization and,
    28–29
Cognitive impairment, use of
  restraints and, 25–26
Collaborative role with another
  mental health worker, 76–77, 89
Commitment, legal obligations of
  psychiatrist in, 62
Community, participation in
  activities contributing to
  improved, 90
Compassion, psychiatric care with,
  82–83
  in emergency situation, 57–60
  in forensic psychiatry, 70
Competence
  of geriatric patients, 24
  to give consent for release of
    confidential information, 40
  legal, psychiatric examination for,
    41, 87

physician, 54, 82–83
    appeals of dispute over, 83
    to practice outside one's
        professional area, 84
Confidentiality, 39–44
    annotations on principle of,
        39–42, 86–88
    basic rule of, 39
    boundary violations of, 7
    in consultations, 41, 86
    after death, 43
    emancipated minors and, 18
    in emergency situation, 62–63
    examinations for legal purposes
        and, 41, 87
    exceptions to protecting patient,
        17–18
    in forensic psychiatry, 71
    with geriatric population, 24
    limits to, legal obligations and, 62
    nonclinical factors affecting, 18,
        42–43
    of nonclinical information, 8
    psychiatric care of children and,
        16–18, 41, 87
    of psychiatric records, 39, 86–87
    release of information, 40, 86
    outside traditional settings, 21
    in treating severe mental illness, 42
Consent, 12. *See also* Informed
    consent
Consultations, xi, 75–77
    circumstances indicating need
        for, 75–76
    confidentiality in, 41, 86
    difference of opinion between
        treating and consulting
        psychiatrists, 76, 88–89
    referring patient for, 76
    request of patient or family for,
        75, 76, 89
Contact, physical, 6–7. *See also*
    Boundary Violations

Continuing education, responsibility
    for, 88
Contractual arrangement, 84
Cost containment, psychiatric care
    of elderly and, 23. *See also*
    Managed care
Countertransference, 19
Court order to release information,
    42, 87
Criminal acts, psychiatric evaluation
    of person charged with, 66–67, 88

Dangerousness standard
    confidential information revealed
        due to, 41–42, 87
    shift toward, 30–31
Death, confidentiality of psychiatric
    information after, 43
Deception, duty to report colleagues
    engaging in, 51–55
Decision-making capacity,
    competence of geriatric patient
    and, 24
Developmental risks of mental
    disorder versus long-term use of
    psychotropics, 15
Diagnosis, psychiatric, 59–60, 61
Dignity, respect for human, 82–83,
    87, 91
    in emergency situation, 57–60
    in forensic psychiatry, 70
Directiveness, 8. *See also* Autonomy,
    patient
Dispute over physician competency,
    appeals available in, 83
Divorced birth parents, informed
    consent for children of, 13
Doctor/patient relationship. *See*
    Therapeutic relationship
Domestic violence, forgoing obligation
    to be honest with patient in cases
    of, 61. *See also* Child abuse; Elder
    abuse and neglect

Dreams, self-disclosure of, 5
Dual relationships, danger of, 4
Duty to report colleagues engaging
    in fraud or deception, 51–55
Duty to warn, 42. *See also*
    Dangerousness standard

Elder abuse and neglect, 24, 25, 62
Elderly, psychiatric care of. *See*
    Geriatric populations
Emancipated minors, informed
    consent of, 13, 14, 18
Emergency care, ethics of, 57–64
    compassion and respect for
        human dignity, 57–60
    confidentiality, 62–63
    honesty with patients and
        colleagues, 60–61
    managed care and, 34
    obligation to treat patients, 64
    psychiatric diagnosis and, 59–60, 61
    respect for law, 61–62
Employee Retirement Income
    Security Act of 1974 (ERISA), 33
Employing one's patient, 7
Enforcement of ethical practice in
    forensic psychiatry, 70–72
Expert, physician role as, 90
Expertise, practicing outside one's, 84
    forensic evaluations, 70

Families and children, psychotherapy
    with, 18–20
Family of child patient, boundary
    violations with, 20
Fantasies, self-disclosure of, 5
Fear of patient, physician, 75–76
Fee-splitting, 85
Financial incentives/penalties
    limiting provision of appropriate
        treatment, informing patient
        of, 92
    in managed care, 36, 37

Financial relationships, avoiding, 7–8
Food and Drug Administration
    approved versus unlabeled uses
        of psychotropic medication, 14
*Forced Into Treatment: The Role of
    Coercion in Clinical Practice*
    (Group for the Advancement of
    Psychiatry), 28–29
Forensic psychiatry, 65–73
    boundary issues in, 69
    codes of ethics for, 68
    conflict with therapeutic
        relationship and, 69
    definition of, 65
    enforcement of ethical practice
        in, 70–72
    ethical theory in, 66–67
    justice and, 66, 67
Foster care children, 13–14
Fraud, duty to report colleagues
    engaging in, 51–55
Freedom of choice
    patient, 77
    physician, 64, 89–90
Freud, Sigmund, 1
Fund-raising activities, 9

Geriatric populations, 23–26
    competence and consent of, 24
    confidentiality with, 24
    elder abuse and neglect, 24, 25, 62
    insurance coverage of, 23
    quality of life of, 25
    research on, 26
    restraints, use of, 25–26
Gifts, 5–6, 45–50
    cost and nature of, 46–47
    from industry, 48–49
    from patients, 6, 45–47
    reasons behind giving, 46, 47
Government. *See also* Law
    advising and consulting with
        branches of, 90

powers of, 30, 31
Group for Advancement of
    Psychiatry, 28–29
Guidelines
    AMA Code of Medical Ethics,
        48
    APA Code of Medical Ethics, 54
    for forensic psychiatry (AAPL),
        68–69, 71–72
    managed care
        discussion of, 33
        guidelines for dealing with
            managed care (AMA),
            35–36
        Guidelines for Ethical Practice
            in Organized Settings and
            Managed Care (APA),
            91–92
        guidelines of practice for
            managed care reviewers
            (APA), 36–37
        Sabin's credo for ethical
            managed care in mental
            health practice, 37–38
    Principles of Medical Ethics, The
        (AMA), x, 81–82
    *Principles of Medical Ethics With
        Annotations Especially
        Applicable to Psychiatry, The*
        (APA), x, 79–92
    Specialty Guidelines for Forensic
        Psychologists, 68

Harm to self/others, threat of
    patient's, 17. *See also*
    Dangerousness standard
Health insurance. *See* Insurance;
    Managed care
Hippocrates, x, 3, 8
Hippocratic oath, 1, 3
Honesty with patients and
    colleagues, 84–85
    in emergency situation, 60–61
    in forensic psychiatry, 70

Hospitalization
    of children, 21–22
    forgoing obligation to be honest
        with patient in cases of,
        60 61
    involuntary, 27–32, 62

Illegal activity, physician, 85
Illness, self-disclosure of, 5
Impaired physicians' committees,
    54
Impairment
    cognitive, use of restraints and,
        25–26
    reporting physician, 51–55
Industry, gifts from, 48–49
Infant psychiatry, 11. *See also*
    Children, psychiatric care of
Influencing patient, avoidance of,
    8–9
Information
    available in treatment situation,
        use of, 8, 84
    for patient to make informed
        treatment decisions, 33–34,
        35, 92
    release of, 40, 86
        court order for, 42, 87
Informed consent
    competence of geriatric patients
        and, 24
    full disclosure of material
        information, 33–34, 35, 92
    psychiatric care of children and,
        12–14
    for release of confidential
        information, 40, 86
Injury, self-disclosure of, 5
Insurance. *See also* Managed care
    confidentiality issues and, 18,
        42–43
    coverage of geriatric populations,
        23

Intent to harm others, patient's, 17.
    See also Dangerousness
    standard
Involuntary hospitalization, 27–32, 62
    coercion and, 28–29
    criteria for, 27
    ethics principles for, 27–28
    law and, 29–32
    severe mental illness and, 30
Involuntary treatment, 90
    outpatient, 31–32

Justice, 66
    ethical theory of forensic
        psychiatry based on, 67

"Kendra's law," 32

Law
    confidentiality exceptions based
        on statutes, 18
    forensic psychiatry and ethics of
        adversarial legal system, 67
    involuntary hospitalization and,
        29–32
    mandated reporting of physician
        impairment, 51, 54
    respect for, 85
        in emergency situation, 61–62
Legal authority to give informed
    consent for children, 13–14
Legal purposes, psychiatric
    examination for, 41, 87
Libertarianism, opposition to
    involuntary treatment based on,
    28
Litigants, forensic evaluation of, 66–67

Managed care, 33–38
    alternative treatments and,
        33–34, 35
    AMA guidelines for dealing with,
        35–36

APA guidelines of practice for
    managed care reviewers,
    36–37
confidentiality issues and, 42–43
defining, 33–34
effects on medical practice, 34–35
Guidelines for Ethical Practice in
    Organized Settings and
    (APA), 91–92
    review process, 92
hospitalization of children and,
    21
patient advocacy and, 35
Sabin's credo for ethical, in
    mental health practice,
    37–38
Media information on misconduct,
    reporting, 53
Medical illness, behavioral symptoms
    caused by, 59–60, 61
Medical necessity criteria,
    hospitalization of children and,
    21
Medical records of children, legal
    authority of parents to review or
    obtain copy of, 18
Medicine, forensic psychiatry as
    branch of, 66
Mental illness, severe
    confidentiality issues in treating,
    42
    state legislatures on involuntary
        hospitalization, 30
Mentally ill psychiatrist, interceding
    with, 84
Metabolic rates of children,
    psychotropic drug use and,
    14–15
Mill, John Stuart, 28
Minor, treatment of. See Children,
    psychiatric care of
Missed appointment, charging for,
    84

Neglect, elder, 24, 25
New York City Health and Hospitals Corporation, 31
New York Civil Liberties Union, 31
Nonmaleficence, principle of, 66
Nonsexual boundary violations, 4–9

Obligation to treat patients in emergency, 64
Office of Ethics and Professional Responsibility (APA), xi
On Liberty (Mill), 28
Opinions and Reports of Council on Ethical and Judicial Affairs of AMA, 80
Organized settings, guidelines for ethical practice in, 91–92. *See also* Managed care
Outpatient involuntary treatment, 31–32

Parens patriae power, 30, 31
Parents. *See also* Children, psychiatric care of
confidentiality with adolescent patient and, 16–17
custody
certification and, 61
psychiatric diagnosis and, 59
psychiatric examination and, 41
informed consent for psychiatric care of children, 12–13
stepparents, 13
Participation in activities contributing to improved community, 90
Paternalism, 8, 24, 28
Patient advocacy, managed care and, 35
Peer review of physician competence, 54, 83
Personal observation of misconduct, reporting, 53

Pharmaceutical industry, gifts from, 48–49
Physical contact, 6–7. *See also* Boundary Violations
Physician competence, 54, 83, 84
Physician impairment, reporting, 51–55, 84
Police power, 30, 31
Preschool children, psychotropic medications for, 15
Presentation of patient to scientific gathering/public gathering, 40, 87
Principles of Medical Ethics, The (AMA), x, 81–82
Principles of Medical Ethics With Annotations Especially Applicable to Psychiatry, The (APA), x, 79–92
annotations, 82–90
on confidentiality, 39–42, 86–87
on emergency care, 57–64
on forensic psychiatry, 70–71
Guidelines for Ethical Practice in Organized Settings, 91–92
principles, 81–82
on reporting physician impairment, 51–55, 84
on sexual boundary violations, 3, 84, 88
Privacy, patient waiving of privilege of, 40, 86
Professional courtesy, 89
Professionals, information of colleague misconduct from, 53
Psychiatric diagnosis, caution in applying, 59–60, 61
Psychiatric Ethics (Bloch et al), 29
Psychiatric records, confidentiality of, 39, 86–87

Psychopharmacology, children and, 14–16
  metabolic rates and, 14–15
  secret administration of medication, 15
Publications of board findings of misconduct, reporting, 53

Quality of life, geriatric patients, 25

Rapport, self-disclosure and decrease in, 5
Records
  medical, of children, 18
  psychiatric, 39, 86–87
Referring patients for treatment, counseling, or rehabilitation, 88–89
Release of information, 40
  authorization of patient for, 40, 86
  court order for, 42, 87
  relevant material only, 42, 87
Reporting
  of colleagues engaging in fraud or deception, 51–55
  legal obligations of psychiatrist, 17–18, 62
Research
  clinical researchers, 66
  on geriatric population, 26
  with human subjects, 87
Residency, ethics education during, xiv, 20–21
Respect for human dignity, 82–83, 87, 91
  in emergency situation, 57–60
  in forensic psychiatry, 70
Respect for law, 29–30, 85
  in emergency situation, 61–62
Restraints, use of, 25–26
Reye's syndrome, 15
Right to refuse treatment, 59

Sabin's credo for ethical managed care in mental health practice, 37–38
Sanctions, xi
School-age children, psychotropic medications for, 15
Second opinions, 75–77. See also Consultations
Security purposes, psychiatric examination for, 41, 87
Self-disclosure, 4–5
Self-regulation, responsibility for, 52
Sexual boundary violations, 3–4, 84
  with child patient, 20
Sexual involvement between faculty/ supervisor and trainee/student, 88
Socializing with child patient and/or family, 20, 21
Statutes and regulations. See Law
Stepparents, 13
Supervisory role with another mental health worker, 76–77, 85, 88, 89
Surgeon General of United States, on efficacy of psychiatric treatment, 29

Teaching, clinical information used in, 40, 86
Teaching hospitals, financial viability of, 21–22
Technology, confidentiality and advances in, 18, 40
Tetracycline, 15
Therapeutic frame, 1–2
Therapeutic relationship, 33–34
  boundaries of, 1–2, 83. See also Boundary violations
  conflict with forensic psychiatry and, 69
  gift-giving and, 47

preservation of optimal
    conditions for, 89
Third-party payers, confidentiality
    issues and, 18, 42–43. *See also*
    Managed care
Touching a patient, precautions in,
    6–7. *See also* Boundary Violations
Traditional settings, psychotherapy
    with child patient outside, 20–21
Transference, gift-giving and, 47
Treatment Advocacy Center, 30
Treatment and treatment options
    appropriateness of, 92

managed care and, 33–34, 35
    right to refuse, 59, 77

Utilitarian principle, involuntary
    treatment based on, 27–28

Valproic acid, 15
Violence, domestic, 61. *See also*
    Child abuse; Elder abuse and
    neglect

Writing, clinical information used in,
    40, 86